Demystifying Qualitative Research
in Pregnancy and Childbirth

Demystifying Qualitative Research in Pregnancy and Childbirth

edited by
Tina Lavender, Grace Edwards and Zarko Alfirevic

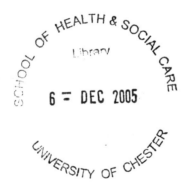
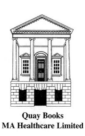

Quay Books
MA Healthcare Limited

Quay Books Division, MA Healthcare Limited, Jesses Farm, Snow Hill, Dinton,
Salisbury, Wiltshire, SP3 5HN

British Library Cataloguing-in-Publication Data
A catalogue record is available for this book

ISBN 185642 259 3

Printed in the UK by Cromwell Press, Trowbridge, Wiltshire

Contents

List of contributors

Tina Lavender (PhD, MSc, RM, RGN) is a Professor of Midwifery and Women's Health at the University of Central Lancashire with an honorary contract at Liverpool Women's Hospital NHS Trust. Tinalav@yahoo.co.uk

Grace Edwards (PhD, MEd Cert. Ed, ADM, RM, RGN) is a Consultant midwife at Liverpool Women's Hospital NHS Trust and Liverpool and Sefton Public Health Network and Lecturer in Midwifery Research at the University of Central Lancashire. Grace.Edwards@lwh-tr.nwest.nhs.uk

Zarko Alfirevic (MD, MRCOG) is a Professor in Fetal and Maternal Medicine at Liverpool University and Liverpool Women's Hospital. zarko@liverpool.ac.uk

Fiona Dykes (PhD, MA, RM, RGN, ADM, CertEd) is a Reader in Maternal and Infant Health and leads the Maternal and Infant Nutrition and Nurture Stream, Midwifery Studies Research Unit, University of Central Lancashire. fcdykes@uclan.ac.uk

Carol Kingdon (MA Distinction, BA Honours) is Research Fellow in the Midwifery Unit, University of Central Lancashire. Carol.kingdon@lwh-tr.nwest.nhs.uk

Donal Manning (MD, FRCPCH, DCH, DRCOG, MSc) is a Consultant paediatrician, Wirral Hospital NHS Trust; Chair of Wirral LREC and member of North West MREC. Donal.manning@whnt.nhs.uk

Jane Morgan (MA, ADM, Cert Ed, RM, RGN) is a Senior Lecturer Midwifery and Research, Edge Hill College. morganj@edgehill.ac.uk

Denis Walsh (MA, PG DipEd, DPSM, RM, RGN) is an Independent Midwifery Lecturer and Midwifery PhD student, University of Central Lancashire. Denis.walsh@ntlworld.com

Lisa Baker (PgDip, RM, RGN) is a practice development midwife at Liverpool Women's Hospital NHS Trust and MPhil student Liverpool University. lisabaker@cbaker.freeserve.co.uk

Claire Snowdon (MA) Research Fellow, London School of Hygiene and Tropical Medicine. cms1000@cam.ac.uk

Diana Elbourne (PhD) Professor of Health Care Evaluation, London School of Hygiene and Tropical Medicine. diana.elbourne@lshtm.ac.uk

Jo Garcia (MSc) Research Fellow, Social Science Research Unit, Institute of Education, London. J.Garcia@ioe.ac.uk

Bernie Carter (PhD, PGCE, BSc, RSCN, SRN) is Professor of Children's Nursing, University of Central Lancashire. bcarter@uclan.ac.uk

Helen Smith (PhD, MA, BA) is a Research Associate, Effective Health Care Alliance Programme. cjdhel@liv.ac.uk

Yana Richens (MSc, BSc, RM, RGN, SEN) is Consultant Midwife in Public Health, University College London Hospital. yana.richens@uclh.org

Lynne Currie (BSc Hons, Dip.App. Soc. Sci) is a researcher for the quality Improvement Programme and a PhD student at the RCN Institution.

Foreword

Good clinical research is recognised today as an essential complement to good clinical practice. Without advances in knowledge, practice stagnates, mistakes are perpetuated, and benefits are denied to those who justifiably assume that their professional advisers question accepted wisdom and seek innovation.

In the past, good clinical care could be maintained by adopting the best practices of previous generations and adapting to changing circumstances. As science and technology advanced, there became increasing need for clinical research to validate current practices and proposed developments. Early randomised trials were usually not powerful enough to yield significant conclusions. However, statistical analysis of the combined results of available randomised trials (meta-analysis) has provided important insights into what works and what does not. The prenatal use of corticosteroids is the best example of an effective treatment long under-used, because of the absence of adequate validation of its effects. In the last twenty years, there has been a great increase in the reporting of large, powerful, clinical trials, many of which have changed the ways in which women and their babies are now cared for during pregnancy and childbirth. Quantitative clinical research has had real impact in our specialties, and will continue to do so. Qualitative research, which is often related to perceptions and to matters of personal choice, has emerged more recently, and is less well understood.

The choice of research method is dictated by the research question, and both quantitative and qualitative approaches require intellectual and methodological rigour. Alone, neither form of research provides the big canvas. For example, the clinical benefits and hazards of planned caesarean section in the absence of clear clinical indication (currently a contentious issue) might be determined by quantitative randomised trials, allowing that ethical and feasibility considerations were appropriate. Qualitative research, on the other hand, could be used to analyse some of the issues influencing women who request Caesarean operations. These issues are complex and include their own personal safety, the perceived safety of their babies, the mothers' wishes and understandings, cultural influences, their need for personal control, and their willingness to delegate decision making to others.

Both of us have had the good fortune to work in a maternity unit where the research (and clinical) contributions of obstetricians and midwives are equally valued, but there are those within the maternity services who see quantitative research as 'hard' and doctor-driven, while they envisage qualitative research as 'soft' and midwife-dominated. Those are myths that this excellent book seeks to dispel. It is timely, and informs clinicians and researchers about the rationale for, and the tools of, qualitative research methods. We believe that this book will help to break down barriers, where they exist, between obstetricians and midwives on concepts of what makes for good research in maternity care.

Dame Lorna Muirhead, Immediate Past-President, Royal College of Midwives
Professor Jim Neilson, Professor of Obstetrics and Gynaecology,
University of Liverpool
Liverpool, August 2004

Introduction

Having been heavily criticised in the seventies for lack of 'evidence base', our speciality has made great strides in embracing the concept of evidence-based clinical practice. One can, therefore, appreciate why most of us constantly bombarded with clear hypotheses, thousands of participants and objective, measurable outcomes may find it difficult to acknowledge the relevance of studies containing a broad research focus, half a dozen participants and findings which are not, and were never intended to be, generalisable. Yet with the growing desire to explore quality of care, as opposed to just quantity, this methodological approach has now been recognised as an integral method of inquiry in maternity care. In fact, the conception of this book followed repeated requests for guidance from midwives and doctors wishing to conduct a piece of qualitative research in a rigorous way and not being able to find a suitable textbook.

We are heartened that the need for qualitative research is no longer forcefully challenged within practice settings. Clinicians do, however, continue to struggle with aspects of qualitative methodology, particularly in terms of theoretical underpinning, data collection and qualitative analysis and few have either the time or the inclination to wade through numerous textbooks that are often written in an unfamiliar language and leave them more confused than when they started!

The information in this book is not exhaustive, but aims to guide readers through all stages of the research process. The journey through the chapters will enlighten them to the purpose of qualitative research; inform them of considerations before they commence any research; outline the theoretical underpinning of the approach; highlight important ethical issues; discuss different methods of data collection; explore the process of analysis; suggest ways of assessing qualitative research; demonstrate how to integrate qualitative and quantitative research; and provide examples of how to explore the views of those who are hard to reach. Pivotal to this information are real research examples from maternity settings, which readers can relate to.

We hope that for those on the first rung of the qualitative research ladder, the information provided will allow their ideas to become a reality. Readers with qualitative research experience can use this book as a foundation from which they will develop more in-depth studies. But for all, the book should be a code-breaker, which has unravelled the complexities of an approach, which has previously mystified many.

Tina Lavender, Grace Edwards and Zarko Alfirevic
May 2004

Chapter 1

Why carry out qualitative research?

Carol Kingdon

> *The method consists in an attempt to build a bridge between*
> *the world of sense and the world of science.*
>
> Bertrand Russell, 1872–1970

Introduction

A knowledge of qualitative research is becoming increasingly important in healthcare systems that not only recognise the value of research into clinical outcomes, but also the benefits of understanding healthcare processes from the perspectives of those involved. Midwives and obstetricians seeking to adopt the methods of qualitative research in practice should appreciate that qualitative research has been a field of inquiry in its own right for nearly a century. Qualitative research has separate and distinguished histories in education, social work, communications, psychology, history, organisational studies, medical science, anthropology and sociology (Denzin and Lincoln, 2000).

Within maternity care obstetricians, midwives and service users have been asked to participate in qualitative research studies for many years. During the 1970s, a number of eminent British sociologists used qualitative interviews to explore the impact of social behaviours and circumstances on maternal and infant health in both the antenatal and postnatal periods (Oakley, 1979; Graham and Mckee, 1979). However, it is only within the last decade that a wider acceptance of the clinical relevance of qualitative research has emerged. As a consequence, scientific review processes for research ethics committees, funding bodies and editorial panels now require knowledge of both quantitative and qualitative research approaches.

In their paper published in the *British Journal of Obstetrics and Gynaecology* in 2001, Pope and Campbell (2001) acknowledged that qualitative research is no longer the sole preserve of social scientists. Clinicians from a wide-range of medical specialities should increasingly accept the methods of qualitative inquiry, such as in-depth interviews, focus groups and observation. Only six years earlier, the *British Medical Journal* ran a series of articles by the same authors introducing qualitative research to a largely uninitiated medical audience (Pope and Mays, 1995; Mays and Pope, 1995a, 1995b). The articles were commissioned, not as papers about qualitative research, but as a series on 'non-quantitative methods' (Pope and Mays, 1999). This is illustrative of the status and legitimacy accorded to only quantitative research in many medical specialties at the time.

In the past, the distinction between 'hard' and 'soft' data, and talk of a quantitative/qualitative divide has exacerbated the view that qualitative research is in some way inferior to quantitative (Rees, 2003). Where a quantitative/qualitative divide still exists it is a false polarisation, compounded by the promotion of hierarchies of evidence within which qualitative research has no place. Miller and Crabtree (2000: 612–3) state:

> *Evidence-based medicine is the new wonder child in clinical care and in clinical research. The proliferation of clinical practice guidelines is one result of these initiatives. Another result is the relative reduced value of qualitative studies. But evidence-based medicine actually offers qualitative clinical investigators multiple opportunities — there is so much missing evidence!*

Evidence from qualitative research alone is not the only way clinical researchers can 'discover' all this missing evidence. The findings of qualitative and quantitative research undertaken either concurrently or consecutively can compliment each other to aid understanding of the bigger picture. Undertaken alongside quantitative research, qualitative research may contribute to the evidence-based healthcare agenda by enhancing understanding of why interventions work; improving the accuracy and relevance of quantitative studies; identifying appropriate variables to be studied in quantitative research; offering explanations for unexpected results from quantitative work; and by generating hypotheses to be tested using quantitative methods (Black, 1994).

There are also important ways 'in which qualitative research can contribute to the pursuit of evidence based healthcare that are independent of the contribution of other methodologies' (Popay and Williams, 1998: 34). Popay and Williams (1998) discuss important examples of qualitative research that have explored 'taken for granted' practices in health care. They cite the work of Goffman (1961) as a particularly dramatic illustration of how qualitative research can show how healthcare institutions affect the behaviour of people that live and work within them. Goffman's observations of a single ward contributed to a paradigm shift in mental healthcare policy that has resulted in more humane, appropriate, effective and efficient care provision. Popay and Williams (1998) also discuss the value of 'stand-alone' qualitative research in offering a 'difference model' to understand lay/clinical behaviour, patient's perceptions of quality/ appropriateness of care, organizational culture, change management and the evaluation of complex policy initiatives.

This chapter highlights the relevance of qualitative traditions to the study of everyday maternity care processes, the appropriateness of methods of qualitative inquiry to particular research questions, and the increasing value of qualitative research for maternity care policy makers. The intention is to lay the foundations for the book as a whole by defining the place for using (or not using) the methods of qualitative inquiry for the benefit of future evidence-based care. The use of examples from contemporary research investigating rising Caesarean section rates is intended to both illustrate key points and to establish the place of qualitative research in the study of this global phenomenon. A variety of exemplar qualitative studies investigating the medicalisation of birth, and interaction and communication in the intrapartum period are also cited to demonstrate how qualitative research can influence maternity care practice at individual, organisational and policy levels.

The chapter is divided into six key sections:

- what is qualitative research
- qualitative research to understand everyday processes
- qualitative research and healthcare policy
- the impact of qualitative research on practice
- qualitative research to complement randomised controlled trial methodology

- qualitative research and consumer involvement.

The first section discusses the defining characteristics of qualitative research and why a single homogeneous definition of 'qualitative research' remains so elusive.

What is qualitative research?

Murphy *et al* (1998) introduce qualitative research as a process that involves the collection, analysis and interpretation of data that are not easily reduced to numbers. Langford (2001) provides an equally succinct definition, describing qualitative research as an objective process used to examine subjective human experiences by using non-statistical methods of analysis. However, defining qualitative research as the antithesis to quantitative is helpful only at a very basic level. Because as acknowledged by Pope and Campbell (2001: 233) when posing exactly the same question: 'What is qualitative research? The answer varies depending on whom you ask.'

Sociologists working within social action theory, symbolic interactionism, phenomenology and ethnomethodology have traditionally used the methods of qualitative research (semi-structured interviews or participant observation) to acquire data rich in depth and meaning about individuals and social groups. Anthropology is a separate discipline to sociology, with anthropologists characteristically using ethnography in their fieldwork. Ethnography has evolved as 'multi-method' qualitative research that usually includes observation, participation, archival analysis and interviewing, thus combining the assets and weakness of each method (Reinharz, 1992). Fiona Dykes discusses research paradigms and the methodologies of the respective disciplines in more detail in the next chapter. The key point for this chapter is to recognise that 'qualitative research' has separate and distinguished histories within many social science disciplines. Those planning to undertake qualitative studies would benefit from understanding the wide choice of theoretical traditions, methodological approaches and methods of collecting data available to them.

Across the many disciplines engaged in qualitative research in the past or present, there is no single all encompassing homogeneous definition of 'qualitative research', so I have selected the following two extracts from the first and second editions of Denzin and Lincoln's edited collection the *Handbook of Qualitative Research* (1994; 2000) for the purpose of this chapter. The quotes emphasise many of what I believe to be the defining characteristics of qualitative research:

> *The word qualitative implies an emphasis on the qualities of entities and on processes and meanings that are not experimentally examined or measured (if measured at all) in terms of quantity, amount, intensity, or frequency. Qualitative researchers stress the socially constructed nature of reality, the intimate relationship between the researcher and what is studied, and the situational constraints that shape inquiry.*

Denzin and Lincoln, 2000: 8

> *Qualitative research is multi-method in focus, involving an interpretive,*
> *naturalistic approach to its subject matter. This means that qualitative*
> *researchers study things in their natural settings, attempting to make sense*
> *of or interpret phenomena in terms of the meanings people bring to them.*
> *Qualitative research involves the studied use and collection of a variety of*
> *empirical materials — case study, personal experience, introspective, life*
> *story, interview, observational, historical, interactional, and visual texts-that*
> *describe routine and problematic moments and meaning in individuals' lives.*

(Denzin and Lincoln 1994:2).

In the context of my own work investigating women's views of different ways of giving birth in the light of suggestions of the need for a randomised controlled trial of planned Caesarean section versus planned vaginal birth; qualitative research offers an approach to studying rising Caesarean section rates grounded in the complex interactions between expectant parents, well-intentioned midwives and obstetricians, organisational protocols, cultural norms and the influence of the media, family and friends. The extract below is from a transcript of an interview conducted postnatally with a twenty-eight-year-old woman who had an elective Caesarean section after her baby was diagnosed in the breech position. The extract illustrates the complex reality for this woman in a society where intervention in the physiological processes of birth is perceived by many to have improved on nature, and Caesarean section is no longer reserved for acute obstetric emergencies. Statistics highlighting the global trend towards rising Caesarean section rates tell us about the increasing frequency of the operation, but cannot provide all of the information as to why. The fact that qualitative research is grounded in every day social and cultural interactions is the single most distinguishing characteristic and its greatest strength.

Women's views of different ways of giving birth

This is an extract from a postnatal interview transcript with a twenty-eight-year-old woman whose first baby was delivered by elective Caesarean section during 2002. The interview was conducted as part of my current study exploring a cohort of women's views of different ways of giving birth in both the antenatal and postnatal period.

Carol: Can you tell me how you feel about your childbirth experience?
Helen: Well I think, think it was excellent. It erm... well it was strange really because I came [to the hospital]. I think when we first spoke [first antenatal interview] I really wanted to look at the idea of having a Caesarean. I mean it scared me but... erm. I've heard so many older women talk about having, you know giving birth, loosing their sort of tightness underneath, and erm, becoming incontinent. You even see adverts on the TV with people who've got, pads for women who leak, erm I don't want to have that, I just don't want it.
It was about the time Posh Spice[1] and all that were having Caesareans, too posh to push. Everything was negative, negative Caesarean, you know, major operation. Even in all the, I had my head in a pregnancy magazine every minute

1. 'Posh Spice' Victoria Beckham was one of several high profile celebrities to receive widespread media attention in the UK during 2001 after the birth of their first child by elective Caesaran section

of the day and it was all women who'd had Caesareans, stomach was ruined after it, couldn't push the pram, couldn't breast feed, couldn't bond because they hadn't had a proper natural delivery. I used to think oh my goodness, this is a nightmare. You know it was like, as if you haven't gone through a proper twenty hours of hell, you haven't had like, it's like you haven't given, done what's right as a woman. I think that's stupid really.

Anyway at the time I remember thinking, oh no I'll go for a natural delivery, and it's weird. You know a lot of the reasons for wanting a section as well. My sister's son, I don't know if you remember me telling you? My sister's son is autistic, has learning difficulties and he got into a lot of distress during my sister's labour. My mam, put that down to a bad labour and that's always been in my mind...

But, anyway, it turns that when she turned breech, when it came to about three, four weeks before she was due, the midwife said I don't think you're baby's in the right position here. So they sent me to the clinic, I remember coming back from the midwife, lying in bed and Peter [husband] come in and I was crying. It was a nightmare, this isn't what I wanted I'd finally got my head round having a natural delivery and then when she was breech. They said they'd try and turn the baby, but I didn't want that, we agreed that was how it was meant to be.

Qualitative research to understand everyday processes

One of the most demonstrative examples of the value of qualitative research's *a priori* approach grounded in philosophical assumptions of interpretive and naturalistic enquiry in a contemporary maternity care setting is a qualitative study by Harris and Greene (2002a). The aim of Harris and Greene's (2002a) work was to investigate communication and interaction between midwives, doctors and parents within a single delivery room in Plymouth, UK. The care of twenty women was observed using a ceiling mounted unobtrusive audio-video recorder.

The research findings have been presented at a number of national conferences and study days in the UK (Harris and Greene, 2002a; Harris and Greene, 2002b). From over 111 hours of recording of the first stage and twelve hours recording of the second stage of labour, short video clips of the raw qualitative data frequently have a strong visual impact on audiences presented with the 'reality' of care in units where one-to-one midwifery care equates to midwives spending only 9% of their time supporting women during the first stage of labour.

Harris and Greene's (2002a) study is illustrative of the nature and value of qualitative research in a number of different ways. While results based on a sample of only twenty women may not be generalisable in a quantitative sense, they are transferable to other settings. The findings have a strong resonance with the everyday experiences of many professionals that suggest women accessing hospital care frequently feel unsupported in labour. The Cochrane Review of labour support has shown it to be the only known effective intrapartum intervention to reduce Caesarean section rates (Hodnett, 1999). In the UK, where the national Caesarean section rate continues to increase, Harris and Greene's (2002a) findings are clearly relevant.

Harris and Greene's (2002a) data are rich in the experiences of individuals that could not have been accessed in such depth, in any way other than by using qualitative methods. Harris and Greene's research highlights not only the relevance, but also the importance of qualitative research in the study of everyday processes to aid understanding of what is good about current practice and what is not.

Another completed piece of qualitative research by Murphy *et al* (2003) is also illustrative of how an interpretive approach can highlight where maternity service users needs are not currently being met. Figures from the National Sentinel Caesarean Section Audit (Thomas and Paranjothy, 2001) suggest a third of women in British maternity units undergo operative delivery. Murphy *et al* (2003) conducted interviews with a purposive sample of twenty-seven women who had undergone operative delivery in the second stage of labour between January 2000 and January 2002. The research sought to obtain the views of women on the impact of operative delivery in the second stage of labour, to understand women's experience of delivery and how they made sense of what had happened to them. The study found that women reported deficiencies in antenatal preparation, unrealistic birth plans, a limited understanding of the indication for delivery, and insufficient opportunity for detailed personal review, with operative delivery having a noticeable impact on women's views about future pregnancies and preferred mode of future delivery. Murphy *et al* (2003: 1133) concluded:

> *Women consider postnatal debriefing and medical review important deficiencies in current care. Those who experienced operative delivery in the second stage of labour would welcome the opportunity to have later review of their intrapartum care, physical recovery, and management of future pregnancies.*

Harris and Greene (2002a) and Murphy *et al* (2003) have not only used qualitative research to investigate systematically previously missing evidence of women's experiences of maternity care but, in doing so, have also identified inadequacies in the current delivery of that care.

Qualitative research and healthcare policy

In 1998, the UK's government launched the concept of 'clinical governance' and with it a commitment to improving the quality of health care, in terms of both outcome and the experiences of those receiving care (Department of Health [DoH], 1998). Clinical governance has been defined as a policy, which 'aims to integrate all the activities that impact on patient care into one strategy. This involves improving the quality of information, promoting collaboration, team working and partnerships, as well as reducing variations in practice, and implementing evidence-based practice. Clinical governance is an umbrella term for everything that helps to maintain and improve high standards of patient care' (Currie, Morrell and Scrievener, 2003).

Midwives were asking research questions about the quality of information given to women in labour, a decade before the concept of clinical governance was introduced. Kirkham (1991: 118) in her seminal work exploring midwives information-giving during labour, combined the qualitative methods of observation and interviews to develop an 'analysis "grounded" in her data — data that was also the women's experience'. Kirkham discusses how her choice of qualitative methods meant her, 'viewpoint was widened by childbearing women who, during the course of labour and subsequent interview, showed me the importance to them of things I might otherwise have overlooked. Their observations, values and concepts gave me insights that I would not have had as an ordinary working midwife' (Kirkham, 1991: 118).

In recent years, the emerging clinical governance agenda has had a positive impact on the status of qualitative research as there has been an increasing recognition that its methods of inquiry are often the only way to understand both health processes and their influence on health outcomes from the perspectives of those receiving care. Qualitative research enables researchers to ask questions such as, 'what aspects of maternity care are important to women, how does what is important to them vary depending on their circumstances, and why?' Rather than, 'how many women are there?' A key strength of the inductive process used in qualitative research is generalisations are produced from the empirical process, using participants' own categories and concepts, rather than imposing the researchers predetermined categories to test a hypothesis.

Qualitative work undertaken by Weaver (2000: 488) has illustrated the importance of midwives and obstetricians acknowledging 'some of the shared cultural and social understandings of childbearing women: the explanations available to them when they try to make sense of their experiences and the sort of knowledge that is drawn upon when they talk to each other about birth.' Because it is around such talk that expectation and fear can be built, and it is in such talk women frame their experiences of what constitutes good and bad quality of care.

Drawing on data from forty-seven interviews with postnatal women which forms part of a wider study investigating choice and decision making in Caesarean section, Weaver (2000) discusses how women talked about vaginal birth as an ideal; yet positive statements about vaginal birth were often followed by a 'but', with the notion of vaginal birth as desirable held in tension with the notion of vaginal birth as difficult or even hazardous. Women talked about images of vaginal birth likely to end in emergency Caesarean section as illustrated in the verbatim quotes below:

I thought that I would probably have another section. And I guess the main reason for that was I felt that I'd really lost confidence from going through what I'd been through before. And I thought I don't want to go through that again and find myself in the same situation where I end up having another [emergency] section. And I thought the only way I really would have gone through a natural birth is if somebody had been able to say look, you will be able to deliver this baby naturally (pp. 489–490).

I suppose I was influenced by the number of people I know that have had emergency Caesarean. I think there's about four people that I know that have had them within the last year or so. That makes a heck of a difference, 'cos that makes you think, my goodness is this ever going to be possible? Do people actually give birth naturally?

The quotes also demonstrate some of the many ways in which the women justified requesting an elective Caesarean section. Weaver (2000) is cautious about making recommendations from the interview data alone, but feels that her work does highlight areas where changes need to be made. Her study suggests the need to promote positive images of vaginal birth in the management of pregnancy, and for more transparency about the risks associated with Caesarean section. As mentioned earlier in the chapter, qualitative research may not be 'generalisable' in a quantitative sense, but it is transferable and findings that resonate with the experiences of others have the potential to change practice.

The impact of qualitative research on practice

Pope and Campbell (2001: 235) assert 'the best qualitative work — research that is systematic and rigorous — moves beyond common sense, is more than "just anecdote" and has the power to transform clinical practices in positive ways.' In a similar way to that whereby Goffman's work contributed to a paradigm shift in mental health policy, a continuum of qualitative research investigating women's everyday 'taken for granted' experiences of maternity care has been influential in contributing to an international maternity care agenda that now advocates informed choice and woman-centred care.

Collectively the works of Shelia Kitzinger (1962, 1978, 1982) and Ann Oakley (1979, 1980) in the 1970s and early 1980s, Mavis Kirkham's work in the late 1980s, and more recently Robbie Davis-Floyd (1994) amongst others, have influenced both individual women during their pregnancies, and groups of men and women as midwives, obstetricians and healthcare policy makers. It is a triumph of feminist qualitative research that so-called 'soft' outcomes, such as communication and understanding, bonding and attachment, and psychosocial support are all now firmly on the policy agenda in both the UK and the USA.

Individual qualitative research studies can also have local impact, which with appropriate dissemination can lead to widespread change. For example, where two fetuses are identified by ultrasound in early pregnancy, but only one fetus is subsequently seen, the 'condition' has been described as a 'vanished twin'. It has been suggested that of all twin pregnancies identified at an early ultrasound scan, thirty percent will become a 'vanished twin', with the mothers traditionally receiving the same antenatal and postnatal care as if they had only ever experienced a singleton pregnancy. Briscoe and Street's (2003) qualitative research with women who had experienced a 'vanished twin' found that women would like acknowledgement of the pregnancy as having started as two babies and ending with only one.

> *The women felt that their pregnancy loss was dismissed by caregivers and that information, advice and reassurance relating to the event were lacking.*
>
> Briscoe and Street, 2003: 52

In response to the study findings, women are now provided with an information sheet to read and take away with them, which provides answers to the questions raised by women during the course of the research.

Many of the examples of qualitative research cited in this chapter highlight how frequently women view their experiences of care negatively. This is not necessarily associated with poor outcomes, but because they did not receive either sufficient information to prepare them for the physical or psychological impact of childbirth, or adequate information to enable them to make informed decisions and actively participate in their care.

O'Cathain *et al* (2002) undertook a randomised controlled trial (RCT) in thirteen maternity units in Wales in order to assess the effect of leaflets on promoting informed choice in women using maternity services. To understand the social context in which the evidence-based leaflets were used; qualitative research was undertaken alongside, but independent from, the trial (Stapleton, Kirkham and Thomas, 2002). The qualitative research found that the environment had a crucial influence on the way in which the leaflets were disseminated, thus affecting informed choice. Stapleton, Kirkham and Thomas (2002: 422) concluded, 'the culture into which the leaflets were introduced supported existing normative patterns of care and this ensured informed compliance rather than informed choice'. Their work illustrates how undertaking qualitative research at the same time as quantitative research is a useful way to identify potential barriers to the implementation of RCT findings by clinicians and maternity service users.

Qualitative research to complement randomised controlled trial methodology

In the social sciences, undertaking qualitative and quantitative research simultaneously to provide a multi-layered, more valid picture is known as triangulation: 'multiple methods or perspectives may be used for the collection and interpretation of data about a phenomenon, in order to obtain an accurate representation of reality' (Polit and Hunger 1999). The advantages of such an approach have been highlighted recently in Lavender and Chapple's (2003) work commissioned by the Department of Health's Neonatal Taskforce to investigate models of maternity care. The data from the quantitative questionnaire element of the study indicated that the majority of women wanted immediate access to doctors, a Special Care Baby Unit in the place where they give birth, and twenty-four-hour access to epidurals. However, the qualitative data found that that women were clearly unaware that midwives have the ability to work autonomously, identify risk and deal with obstetric emergencies. The triangulation of data suggested women's current beliefs might be misguided by their lack of knowledge about the midwife's role. Issues surrounding the combining quantitative and qualitative data are discussed in detail in *Chapter 7*, so I will consider only briefly the advantages of undertaking qualitative research to complement quantitative data specifically from randomised controlled trials.

Oakley (2000) has described the randomised controlled trial (RCT) as medicines prime way of knowing. The RCT evolved as an alternative to the uncontrolled experimentation of 'normal' practice, and as offering answers to questions about effectiveness and safety, which individual doctors cannot answer from the experience of individual cases (Oakley, 2000). The synthesis of evidence from RCTs using meta-analysis within Cochrane Systematic Reviews began in the field of pregnancy and childbirth. Consequently, the focus on evidence-based practice in obstetrics is well developed (Audit Commission, 1997). It is unfortunate that an unintended consequence of evidence-based practice has been a false polarisation of quantitative and qualitative research, compounded by increasing popularity of a hierarchy of evidence considered worthy of influencing a change in clinical practice.

However, obstetrics and midwifery is more than the application of scientific rules that dictate practice only if based on evidence from RCTs.

Caring for women during pregnancy and birth has a profoundly human element where clinical judgement is also informed by social context. It is widely acknowledged that RCTs are the best source of evidence of the effectiveness of clinical interventions (Popay and Williams, 1998; Miller and Crabtree, 2000) but evidence of effectiveness alone does not necessarily mean that an intervention will be widely implemented:

Miller and Crabtree (2000: 613) have argued:

> *Read any RCT report, the only voice you hear is the cold sound of*
> *intervention and the faint echoes of the investigator's biases. The*
> *cacophonous music of patients, clinicians, insurance companies, lawyers,*
> *government regulatory bodies, consumer interest groups, community*
> *agencies, office staff, corporate interests and family turmoil is mute. There*
> *has also been little research into the clinical expertise side of the EBM*
> *equation and the associated areas of relationship dynamics, communication,*
> *and patient preference: there is much to be learnt about how patients and*
> *clinicians actually implement 'best evidence'.*

Qualitative research can investigate practitioners' and patients' attitudes, beliefs and preferences, and the whole question of how evidence is turned into practice (Green and Britten, 1998: 1230). For example, the UK's Royal College of Obstetricians and Gynaecologists (RCOG) *Clinical Green Top Guidelines on the Management of Breech Presentation* recommend all women with uncomplicated breech presentation at term (thirty-seven to forty-two weeks) should be offered external cephalic version (ECV) (Johanson, 2001: 1). This guideline is based on the results of six RCTs that have found a significant reduction in the risk of Caesarean section in women where there is an intention to undertake ECV without any increased risk to the baby.

There are few published studies evaluating women's views of the procedure, and there is clearly a need for more qualitative research to understand the appropriateness of ECV from the perspective of pregnant women. While ECV is not the focus of my work, investigating women's views of different ways of giving birth, it has been an issue for the women who have participated in the study and their baby has been in the breech position at term. The procedure was clearly not acceptable to 'Helen' quoted earlier (*p. 4*) but we do not know whether this is because of the way information about ECV was provided to her, or whether she viewed elective Caesarean section as less 'risky' than ECV. A collaborative study involving both obstetric and midwifery colleagues at Liverpool Women's Hospital, UK is currently using qualitative interviews to explore why women decline the evidence-based intervention of ECV (Walkinshaw, Blayney and Briscoe, 2004).

Conducting an RCT is a fruitless exercise if the results are not acceptable to women and/or clinicians. Bewley and Cockburn (2002) make reference to a powerful debate taking place in the medical and lay press regarding elective Caesarean section for 'maternal request' even in normal uncomplicated pregnancies. However, as professional concerns promoting physiological birth at one end of the spectrum and Caesarean section at the other are increasingly taking centre stage, there is a danger of losing site of the fundamentally important question of how the individual women accessing contemporary maternity care actually feel about elective Caesarean section in the absence of a clinical indication.

As I have asserted in an earlier publication, 'women's views are pivotal to the debate'. Without knowing whether women feel that elective Caesarean section is acceptable or on what 'evidence' they form their views of delivery mode, the desirability (let alone feasibility) of designing a RCT to construct the quantitative evidence is irrelevant (Kingdon *et al*, 2003). As acknowledged by Boote, Telford and Cooper (2002: 218) in maternity care, in particular, pressure from consumer representative groups has arisen from awareness that interventions have been introduced without sufficient evaluation and without taking the views and reported experiences of women using maternity services into account.

Qualitative research and consumer involvement

In the UK, the National Childbirth Trust (NCT) has actively challenged the medical model of 'passive patient and active doctor' since the 1970s (Oliver, 1995). Boote *et al* (2002: 217) have asserted 'a consumer perspective is important theoretically in any aspect of health care, be it service development, audit or research, because it complements the perspective of the clinician and the biomedical researcher by providing a more holistic interpretation of health as defined by the World Health Organization.'

A number of influential bodies, including the international Cochrane Collaboration, the Consumers' Health Forum of Australia and the UK's Department of Health have all now advocated that the public should have a more participatory role in the processes of health research, with my use of the term 'consumer' consistent with its use by these organisations. However, Boote, *et al*'s Venn diagram for classifying consumers in relation to healthcare (reproduced in *Figure 1.1*) illustrates the complexity of the range of individuals and groups who may be defined by the term.

Many of the advocates of qualitative research within social science disciplines regard the knowledge and practice of trained experts as locally variable, as is the knowledge and practice of lay people. Anthropologists, in particular, typically include both the knowledge and practice of lay and experts within the boundaries of their research (Lambert and McKevitt, 2002). Consequently, both the theoretical concepts underpinning good qualitative research and their methodological application have a natural affinity with the principles of consumer involvement in research.

The opportunities for involving consumers in qualitative research span the spectrum of consumer involvement in research from the identification of topics to the analysis and dissemination of research results. The advantages of involving consumers in qualitative research are multiple. For example, a collaborative qualitative project involving midwives and consumers in Blackburn, UK is currently investigating postnatal depression through interaction with South Asian women (Byrom and Patel, 2003). Focus groups and semi-structured interviews are being used to explore women's experiences of childbirth and pregnancy, their use of maternity and health visiting services and the influence of their family networks and social support. This would would not have been possible without the involvement of members of South Asian community as facilitators and interviewers.

Nearly a decade ago, Chalmers (1995) suggested greater lay involvement in setting the research agenda would almost certainly lead to greater open mindedness about which questions are worth addressing, which forms of health care merit assessment, and which treatment outcomes matter. Greater open mindedness is also required to accept the value of qualitative research to provide answers to such important research questions.

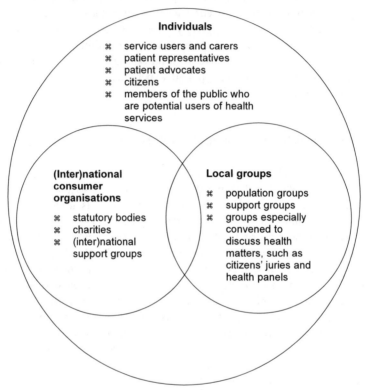

Figure 1.1: Classifying consumers in relation to health care, reproduced with permission from Boote *et al*, 2002: 217

Conclusion – why carry out qualitative research?

Properly designed qualitative research sits comfortably alongside the most rigorous quantitative research and it should not be viewed as an easy substitute for a 'statistical' or quantitative study (Creswell, 1998: 16). For a field that is so well established in the social sciences it is especially unfortunate that 'qualitative research' has so frequently been used in maternity care as a generic term to refer to a variety of studies, of varying quality, collecting non-quantitative data.

Historically, high quality qualitative research has been published by and for other social scientists in a language, and in places, that benefits them. It is unfortunate that so few studies have been widely disseminated to inform the obstetricians or midwives providing maternity care and the individual women accessing this care. However midwives' and doctors' increasing use of social science methodologies has already begun to change this, with exemplar qualitative research increasingly being published in high impact journals with obstetric and midwifery readership.

There are now many excellent examples of qualitative research investigating aspects of contemporary maternity care. *Table 1.1* summarises some of the most pertinent reasons for embarking on a piece of qualitative research. Helen Smith's chapter (*Chapter 9*) discusses in detail the absence of the same depth of knowledge about how to synthesise the findings of qualitative studies as there is for quantitative data (meta-analysis). While opinions vary as to the appropriateness of trying, the standards by which qualitative research is undertaken today will undoubtedly continue to be scrutinised in some form in the future.

Table 1.1: Why carry out qualitative research?	
Qualitiative research can be undertaken to:	**Qualitative research can complement quantitative research by:**
Explore taken for granted practices in health care	Enhancing understanding of why interventions work
Understand health behaviours in their social context	Offering explanations for unexpected results from quantitative work
Investigate perceptions of quality/appropriateness of care	Generating hypotheses to be tested using quantitative methods

Qualitative research should always be conducted to the highest methodological standards applicable if it is to inform future evidence-based care. There are so many unanswered clinical research questions, some of which require quantitative data, while others will be most appropriately addressed with qualitative data, and increasingly complex questions will benefit from research designs that incorporate both. I hope this chapter has demonstrated the relevance and the importance of qualitative research in maternity care to a wider audience — and possibly inspired you to read on and take advantage of the multiple opportunities afforded by so much missing evidence.

Acknowledgements

I would like to thank Gill Gyte for her comments on an earlier draft of this chapter.

Suggested further reading

All of the papers listed below also appear in the list of references for the chapter, but I have selected them specifically as useful starting points.

Green J, Britten N (1998) Qualitative research and evidence-based medicine. *Br Med J* **316**: 1230–32
This short paper uses the example of asthma treatment to introduce naturalism, interpretation, process, interaction, and relativism as the basic orientations of qualitative methods from the perspective of medical sociologists and illustrate how qualitative research can broaden the notion of 'evidence-based medicine'.

Miller WL, Crabtree BF (2000) Clinical research. In: Denzin NK, Lincoln YS, eds. *Handbook of Qualitative Research*. 2nd. edn. Sage Publications, London: 607–31
The second edition of Denzin and Lincoln's edited collection the *Handbook of Qualitative*

Research is a classic text. This paper by Miller and Crabtree uses teh example of the breast cancer drug 'tamoxifen' not only to illustrate the potential of qualitative research, but to push the boundaries of qualitative methods advocating a participatory, collaborative, multi-method approach involving healthcare professionals and consumers.

Murphy E, Dingwall R, Greatbatch D, Parker S, Watson P (1998) Qualitative methods in health technology assessment: a review of the literature. *Health Technol Assessment* **2**(16) Commissioned by the UK's NHS Research & Development Health Technology Assessment Programme this review provides an excellent introduction to qualitative research methods.

Popay J, Williams G (1998) Qualitative research and evidence-based healthcare. *J Roy Soc Med* **91**(supplement 35): 32–7
This paper provides examples of the type of knowledge, and ways of knowing, that means qualitative research can make a unique contribution to evidence-based healthcare. The authors also make a useful distinction between two different models of the potential role of evidence from qualitative research in the assessment of healthcare — an 'enhancement' (in relation to quantitative) model and a 'difference' (standalone) model.

Pope C, Campbell R (2001) Qualitative research in obstetrics and gynaecology. *Br J Obstet Gynaecol* **108**(3): 233–7
This paper provides an easily accessible introduction to qualitative research approaches and uses exemplar examples from maternity care to illustrate the key points

References

Audit Commission (1997) *First Class Delivery: Improving maternity services in England and Wales.* DoH, London
Bewley S, Cockburn J (2002) The unfacts of request Caesarean section. *Br J Obstet Gynaecol* **109**: 597–605
Black (1994) Why we need qualitative research. *J Epidemiol Commun Health* **48**: 425–26
Boote J, Telford R, Cooper C (2002) Consumer involvement in health research: a review and research agenda. *Health Policy* **61**: 213–36
Briscoe L, Street C (2003) "Vanished Twin": An exploration of women's experiences. *Birth* **30**: 47–53
Byrom S, Patel K (2003) *Bringing it back home: service user collaboration in research practice. Women centred research: The human approach.* 6th Annual Midwifery Research Conference, Liverpool
Chalmers I (1995) What do I want from health research and researchers when I am a patient? *Br Med J* **310**: 1315–18
Creswell JW (1998) *Qualitative Inquiry and Research Design.* Sage Publications, Thousand Oaks
Currie L, Morrell C, Scrievener R (2003) *Clinical Governance: an RCN resource guide.* Royal College of Nursing, London
Davis-Floyd R (1994) The technocratic body: American Childbirth as cultural expression. *Soc Sci Med* **38**(8): 1125–40

Denzin NK, Lincoln YS (1994) *Handbook of Qualitative Research*. Sage Publications, London

Denzin NK, Lincoln YS (2000) *Handbook of Qualitative Research*. 2nd edn. Sage Publications, London

Department of Health (1998) *A First Class Service: Quality in the New NHS*. DoH, London

Goffman E (1961) *Asylums: essays on the social situation of mental patients and other inmates*. Anchor, New York

Graham H, McKee L (1979) *The First Months of Motherhood*. Health Education Council, London

Green J, Britten N (1998) Qualitative research and evidence-based medicine. *Br Med J* **316**(16): 1230–2

Harris M, Greene K (2002a) *How good communication and support — or their absence — affect labour outcomes. The rising Caesarean section rate: from audit to action*. Royal College of Physicians, London

Harris M, Greene K (2002b) *Midwifery support in labour: Are we 'with women'? MIDIRS Hot Topic Study Day: Caesarean section: Reversing the trend*. Manchester Conference Centre, Manchester

Hodnett E (1999) *Caregivers Support during Childbirth: Homelike versus Conventional Institutional settings for birth*. Cochrane Library, issue 4. Update Software, Oxford

Johanson RB (2001) *The management of breech presentation — Green Top Guidelines*. Royal College of Obstetricians and Gynaecologists, London

Kingdon C, Lavender T, Gyte G, Cattrell R, Singleton V, Neilson JP (2003) Who's choosing Caesarean section. *Br J Midwif* **11**(6): 391

Kirkham M (1991) Midwives and information-giving during labour. In: Robinson S, Thompson A, eds. *Midwives, Research and Childbirth*. Volume 1. 3rd edn. Chapman and Hall, London

Kitzinger S (1962) *The Experience of Childbirth*. Penguin, London

Kitzinger S (1978) *Giving Birth: The parents' emotions in childbirth*. Schocken Books, New York

Kitzinger S (1982) The social context of birth: Some comparisons between childbirth in Jamaica and Britain. In: MacCormack C, ed. *Ethnography of Fertility and Birth*. Academic Press, New York: 181–204

Lambert H, McKevitt C (2002) Anthropology in health research: from qualitative methods to multi-disciplinarity. *Br Med J* **325**: 210–13

Langford R (2001) *Navigating the Maze of Nursing Research*. Mosby, St Louis

Lavender T, Chapple J (2002) *Models of Maternity care: Midwives and Women's views*. Report for DoH, London

Mays N, Pope C (1995a) Qualitative research: rigour and qualitative research. *Br Med J* **311**: 109–12

Mays N, Pope C (1995b) Qualitative research: observational methods in healthcare settings. *Br Med J* **311**: 182–84

Miller WL, Crabtree BF (2000) Clinical research. In: Denzin NK, Lincoln YS, eds. *Handbook of Qualitative Research*. 2nd edn. Sage Publications, London: 607–31

Murphy DJ, Pope C, Frost J, Liebling RE (2003) Women's views on the impact of operative delivery in the second stage of labour: qualitative interview study. *Br Med J* **327**: 1132

Murphy E, Dingwall R, Greatbatch D, Parker S, Watson P (1998) Qualitative methods in health technology assessment: a review of the literature. *Health Technol Assessment* **2**(16)

Oakley A (1979) *Becoming a Mother*. Martin Robertson, Oxford

Oakley A (1980) *Women Confined*. Martin Robertson, Oxford

Oakley A (2000) *Experiments in Knowing*. Polity Press, Cambridge

O'Cathain A, Walters SJ, Nicholl JP, Thomas KJ, Kirkham M (2002) Use of evidence-based leaflets to promote informed choice in maternity care: randomised controlled trial in everyday practice. *Br Med J*: **324**: 136–44

Oliver S (1995) How can health service users contribute to the NHS Research & Development agenda? *Br Med J* **310**: 1318–20

Pollit DF, Hunger BD (1999) *Nursing Research*. 6th edn. Lippicott, New York

Popay J, Williams G (1998) Qualitative research and evidence-based healthcare. *J Roy Soc Med* **91**(Supplement 35): 32–7

Pope C, Campbell R (2001) Qualitative research in obstetrics and gynaecology. *Br J Obstet Gynaecol* **108**(3): 233–7

Pope C, Mays N (1995) Qualitative research: Reaching the parts other methods cannot reach: an introduction to qualitative methods in health and health services research. *Br Med J*: **311**: 42–5

Pope C, Mays N (1999) *Qualitative Research in Healthcare*. 2nd edn. BMJ Books, London

Reinharz S (1992) *Feminist Methods in Social Research*. Oxford University Press, Oxford

Stapleton H, Kirkham M, Thomas G (2002) Qualitative study of evidence-based leaflets in maternity care. *Br Med J* **324**

Thomas J, Paranjothy S (2001) *The National Sentinel Caesarean Section Audit*. RCOG Press, London.

Walkinshaw S, Blayney S, Briscoe L (2004) Exploration of reasons why women decline the evidence-based intervention of external cephalic version. Unpublished Protocol

Weaver J (2000) Talking about Caesarean section. *MIDIRS Midwif Digest* **10**: 4

Chapter 2

What are the foundations of qualitative research?

Fiona Dykes

*Everything real must be experienceable somewhere, and every kind
of thing experienced must somewhere be real.*
William James, 1842–1910

Introduction

Before a researcher embarks on a research project s/he needs to consider the foundations of qualitative research. This includes understanding what is meant by the terms paradigm, epistemology, ontology and theoretical perspective and knowing how these relate to methodology and method. When submitting qualitative research for publication or a thesis, the author will be expected to make clear her/his connections between, epistemology, ontological position, theoretical perspective and methodology. This chapter aims to assist both readers of research and those actively engaging in research to understand these terms and their implications for the qualitative research process. Examples from maternal and infant health research are provided to assist the reader in connecting theory with practice. It is not the purpose of this chapter to describe the controversial history of the development of qualitative research. Murphy *et al* (1998) provide a useful overview of this in *Health Technology Assessment*.

Paradigms

A useful starting place when focusing on the underpinning assumptions of qualitative research is upon the notion of the paradigm. Kuhn's (1970) revolutionary book, *Structure of Scientific Revolutions*, highlighted that for a given community or discipline there is a specific range of beliefs, values and methods of solving a puzzle. He referred to this way of 'seeing' the world by a specific discipline as a paradigm. The definition of a paradigm has since been somewhat extended from focus upon specific disciplines to emphasis upon the basic human beliefs, world-view and constructions that guide action (Denzin and Lincoln, 1994). This emphasises scope for more individual world-views, rather than homogenising people within a discipline. However, the discipline within which individuals are taught has a strong influence upon the way in which they learn to view the world. A natural scientist may develop a very different way of explaining and trying to understand the world from a sociologist. A person's paradigmatic stance influences what s/he attends to and what is ignored or taken for granted. This relates to Latour's (1987) notion of 'black boxing', involving closing off attention to specific aspects of a phenomenon because they have been 'proven' or established.

Everyone has a paradigmatic stance, whether they are aware of it or not, and this brings with it advantages and disadvantages. A major disadvantage is that it limits people's understandings of others' perspectives. However, there are also advantages, as summarised by Davis-Floyd and St John (1998: 3):

> *Paradigms provide clear conceptual models that facilitate one's movement in the world. In acting not only as models of — but also as templates for — reality, paradigms enable us to behave in organized ways, to take actions that make sense under a given set of principles. To 'paradigm' if you will, is to create the world through the story we tell about it. We then can live as cultural beings in the organized and coherent paradigmatic world we have created. We cannot live without paradigms. But we can learn to be conscious and aware of how they influence our thoughts and shape our experience, to understand that they open some possibilities while closing others. That awareness can bring a rare kind of freedom to 'think beyond'.*

To understand the ways in which two disciplines may differ in their paradigmatic stance, it is useful to simplify the three elements encompassed by a paradigm into epistemology, ontology and methodology. Crotty (1998) provides useful definitions: Epistemology is the 'the theory of knowledge [....] a way of understanding and explaining how we know what we know' (p. 3); ontology is the 'the study of being [....] concerned with "what is", with the nature of existence, with the structure of reality' (p. 10); 'methodology refers to the strategy, plan of action, process or design lying behind the choice and use of particular methods' (p. 3). Put simply, epistemology is 'knowing', ontology is 'being' and methodology relates to the strategy underpinning 'exploration'. Interconnections between these are illustrated in *Figure 2.1*.

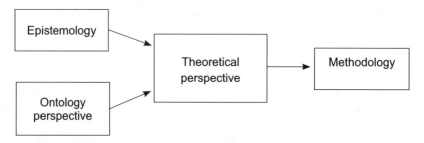

Figure 2.1: Relationships between epistemology, ontology, theoretical perspective and methodology

Knowing and being

To understand the ways in which we 'know' it is useful to compare two contrasting epistemologies: objectivism and constructionism.

Objectivism

Objectivism underpins the theoretical perspective of positivism that constituted the received world view of the emerging natural sciences (Guba and Lincoln, 1994). It may be defined as the:

*View that things exist as meaningful entities independently of consciousness
and experience, that they have truth and meaning residing in them as objects
and that careful research can attain that objective truth and meaning.*

Crotty, 1998: 5, 6

The objectivist epistemology when applied to methodology places emphasis upon testing hypotheses by deduction and providing concrete explanations. Importance is attached to objectivity, control and replicability. This approach inevitably requires quantification and involves the collection and collation of quantitative data. The methodology that is considered to be superior within the objectivist epistemology is experimental with the 'gold standard' being the randomised controlled trial. As this chapter relates to qualitative research, objectivism and quantitative methodologies are not discussed further.

Constructionism

Constructionism emerged as a critique of the objectivist epistemology. In their classic text, *The Social Construction of Reality*, Berger and Luckmann (1967), two of the key originators of constructionism, focused particularly on reality as it is perceived and experienced by 'ordinary members of society' in their everyday lives (p. 33). However, and crucially, they recognised that humans exist within an external world and that they are inextricably linked with that world.

The reality of everyday life is organized around the 'here' of my body and the 'now' of my present. This 'here' and 'now' is the focus of my attention to the reality of everyday life (p. 36).

Crotty (1998: 42) provides a useful summary of constructionism as the:

*View that all knowledge, and therefore all meaningful reality as such,
is contingent upon human practices being constructed in and out of
interaction between human beings and their world, and developed and
transmitted within an essentially social context [....] meaning is not
discovered but constructed.*

The constructionist epistemology is concerned with understanding from others' perspectives, and qualitative methodologies constitute an obvious way of eliciting this data. Mason (1996) illustrates the constructionist researcher's way of 'knowing' and 'being' in that s/he would hold an ontological position that, 'people's knowledge, views, understandings, interpretations, experiences and interactions are meaningful properties of the social reality which [their] research questions are designed to explore' (p. 39). This, Mason continues, would comply with the epistemology that an acceptable way to, 'generate data on these ontological properties is to interact with people, to talk to them, to listen to them and to gain access to their accounts and articulations' (p. 40).

There are a range of theoretical perspectives that enable the constructionist to understand the phenomena being explored; for example, symbolic interactionism, phenomenology, critical theory and feminism. These are returned to in more depth later in this chapter. It is useful to make the distinction between constructionism, as defined here, with its emphasis upon humans as being inextricably linked to the world and constructing meaning through their interactions with aspects of the world, and the ontologically relativistic stance that underpins the theoretical perspectives of postmodernism and post-structuralism. These perspectives are not further referred to in this chapter, but a number of useful texts may be read to assist with understanding, for example: Turner, 1987, 1992; Fox, 1993; Shildrick, 1997; and Kendall and Wickham, 1999.

Theoretical perspectives

Qualitative researchers also need to be clear about their theoretical perspective, ie. 'the philosophical stance informing the methodology' and providing a context for the research process (Crotty, 1998: 3). There are many theoretical perspectives to choose from, each with its own interesting and often controversial history of development. To illustrate the notion of theoretical perspective, four well-used examples are provided: symbolic interactionism; phenomenology; critical theory and feminism. Links between these theoretical perspectives and the methodologies that may be employed are presented in *Table 2.1*.

Table 2.1: Examples of methodologies that relate to specific theoretical perspectives	
Symbolic interactionism	Grounded theory Ethnography
Phenomenology	Phenomenological research
Critical theory	Ethnography (critical) Participative human inquiry Action research
Feminism	Feminist standpoint research

Symbolic interactionsism

Symbolic interactionism is an interpretevist methodology that owes much to the work of Mead (1934), Goffman (1959) and Glaser and Strauss (1967). Blumer (1969) summarises the key tenets of symbolic interactionism arguing that people behave toward 'things' that they encounter 'on the basis of the meanings that these things have for them' (p. 2). The meaning of these things is derived from and arises out of social interactions. Communication occurs through language and other symbols, and through communication people construct symbols. The constructed meanings are 'handled' and 'modified through an interpretive process' (p. 2). Emphasis is placed upon individuals as active, negotiating and interpreting agents in the world rather than them simply being subject to outside influences, although these are acknowledged. Glaser and Strauss (1967) are widely known for translation of the symbolic interactionist perspective into the development of grounded theory, an interpretive methodology that focuses upon negotiated social processes. Symbolic interactionism, in addition to underpinning the methodology of grounded theory, is also deeply embedded within some forms of ethnography (Hammersley and Atkinson, 1995).

Phenomenology

Phenomenology originates in the philosophical writings of Husserl (1931, 1970, 1973). Van Manen (1990: 9) provides a useful summary:

> *Phenomenology aims at gaining a deeper understanding of the nature or meaning of our everyday experiences. Phenomenology asks, 'What is this or that kind of experience like?' It differs from almost every other science in that it attempts to gain insightful descriptions of the way we experience the world pre-reflectively, without taxonomising, classifying, or abstracting it.*

In contrast to symbolic interactionism, Husserlian phenomenology endeavours to bracket off or lay aside the influences of culture and enculturation to expose the human lived experience of a phenomenon in its purest form. However, the Husserlian notion of 'bracketing' has become controversial with other phenomenologists, for example, Heidegger (1962) and Gadamer (1976) developing perspectives that acknowledge that 'experiences can only be understood in terms of one's background, or historicality, and the social context of the experience' (Burke Draucker, 1999: 361). While phenomenology seeks out descriptions and understandings of lived experiences, there are some fundamental differences between theoretical versions of it stemming from different schools of philosophical thought. There are some useful papers written in health journals that highlight the importance of understanding and making explicit one's phenomenological theoretical perspective, for example: Koch, 1995; Walters, 1995; and Burke Draucker, 1999. Phenomenologists conduct phenomenological research, a methodology referred to later in the chapter.

Critical theory

Critical theory is generally associated with the Frankfurt school of critical inquiry and especially the work of Habermas (1972) and a range of political theorists to include Marx, Gramsci and Friere (Kincheloe and McClaren, 1994). Like phenomenology, critical theory in this broad sense has many versions illustrating its contentious history. The definition proposed by Kincheloe and McClaren (1994: 139–40) of a researcher or theorist embracing critical theory, is useful in illustrating the key tenets of this perspective:

> *We are defining a criticalist as a researcher or theorist who attempts to use her or his work as a form of social or cultural criticism and who accepts certain basic assumptions: that all thought is fundamentally mediated by power relations that are social and historically constituted; that facts can never be isolated from the domain of values or removed from some form of ideological inscription; that the relationship between concept and object and between signifier and signified is never stable or fixed and is often mediated by the social relations of capitalist production and consumption; that language is central to the form of subjectivity (conscious and unconscious awareness); that certain groups in any society are privileged over others [....] that oppression has many faces... .*

This perspective stands in sharp contrast with, for example, symbolic interactionism, in that critical theory does not seek simply to understand but to challenge. It moves away from focusing upon interaction and community to centring upon power, conflict, oppression and transformative action (Crotty, 1998). Critical theorists apply their perspective to a range of methodologies, including various forms of participative human inquiry (Reason, 1994), action research (Deery and Kirkham, 2000) and ethnography (Thomas, 1993).

Feminism

Another well established theoretical perspective is feminism. Feminism has evolved through a range of women's movements across the world in response to women's concerns regarding marginalisation in society. Its roots stem from the mobilisation of the Suffrage movement in America and England between 1890 and 1920 (Humm, 1992). In essence, the feminist theoretical perspective centres upon the challenge to dominant assumptions, inequities and social injustice that relate to women. It is critical in the sense that it seeks transformation and emancipation. However, feminism encompasses a diverse range of perspectives that reflect the many phases in its development. Stanley and Wise (1993) provide a useful review and critique of feminist ontology, epistemology and the main developments in feminist thought to include the influences of post-structuralism.

Tong (1998) illustrates the diversities within feminism by producing a typology to illustrate interconnections between feminism and other theoretical perspectives. She devotes a chapter to each of the following: 'liberal feminism', 'radical feminism', 'Marxist and socialist feminism', 'psychoanalytical and gender feminism', 'existentialist feminism', 'post-modern feminism, 'multicultural and global feminism' and 'Eco-feminism'. While many feminists avoid such demarcations, labels do:

> *Signal to the broader public that feminism is not a monolithic ideology,*
> *that all feminists do not think alike, and that, like all other time-honoured*
> *modes of thinking, feminist thought has a past as well as a present and*
> *future. [...] They help mark the range of different approaches, perspectives*
> *and frameworks a variety of feminists have used to shape both their*
> *explanations for women's oppression and their proposed solutions for its*
> *elimination.*

Tong, 1998: 2

The four examples of theoretical perspectives referred to illustrate the diversity within and differences between perspectives that relate to the constructionist epistemology. Having considered one's theoretical perspective, the researcher needs to consider the methodology that s/he intends to employ in order to address the aims of the research.

Selecting the methodology and method

The methodology, defined above, needs to be appropriate to the research aims and coherent with the researcher's theoretical perspective. It influences the research methods selected. Method refers to the 'techniques or procedures used to gather and analyse data related to some research question or hypothesis' (Crotty, 1998: 3). This section provides an outline of several methodologies and the type of methods that may be selected, illustrating each with examples.

Grounded theory

Grounded theory is a methodology that stems from the theoretical perspective symbolic interactionism, referred to above. Grounded theory is frequently utilised in health research with particular reference to the work of Glaser and Strauss (1967) and increasingly, Strauss and Corbin (1990). Like other methodologies the development and uses of grounded theory have generated divergences, contentions and debate and there needs to be some understanding of these issues before adopting the methodology. The following key aspects of grounded theory are drawn from the much quoted Strauss and Corbin (1990) text, *Basics of Qualitative Research: Grounded Theory Procedures and Techniques.* One-to-one interviews or focus groups are commonly employed with data collection and analysis occurring concurrently. This concurrent process involves using early analytical thought generated from initial analysis to generate and test new questions during subsequent data collection. Sampling proceeds throughout the research on the basis of generated concepts that have theoretical relevance to the evolving theory. This is referred to as 'theoretical sampling' (p. 176). A several stage coding procedure is conducted resulting in increasing levels of abstraction and interpretation and the development of clear interconnections between concepts and categories. The researcher engages in a process of collapsing, merging, refining and verifying the generated categories throughout the research process until no further categories emerge, there is no further movement between them and the relationships between categories is well established. This process is referred to as 'theoretical saturation' (p. 188). A central and unifying core category is developed that integrates the other categories.

Two examples of studies are provided to illustrate the use of grounded theory methodology (*Boxes 2.1* and *2.2*). These grounded theory studies explored aspects of adaptation to motherhood within differing contexts. The grounded theories generated support understanding of basic social processes and ways in which the experience of motherhood may be enhanced or hindered.

This analysis of the conceptualisation of early motherhood enabled recommendations to be made for midwives and nurses in supporting women through this experience. The authors describe the methodology utilised for this study in more detail in a related paper (Rogan *et al*, 1997).

Ethnography

Ethnography as a methodology originates from anthropology. As Murphy *et al* (1998) state, social anthropology may be seen as the 'first institutionalised research-led social science in Britain' (p. 39). Ethnography is informed and infused by the notion of culture and enculturation. Helman (1994: 2–3) states:

> *Culture can be seen as an inherited 'lens' through which the individual*
> *perceives and understands the world that he inhabits, and learns how to live*
> *within it. Growing up within any society is a form of enculturation, whereby*

the individual slowly acquires the cultural lens of that society.

The notion of culture then clearly connects with the methodology. As Aamodt (1991: 41) states:

> *Ethnography is a way of collecting, describing and analysing the ways in which human beings categorise the meaning of their world. [....] It attempts to learn what knowledge people use to interpret experience and mould their behaviour within the context of their culturally constituted environment.*

Despite the centrality of culture, ethnography has followed a long and changing journey from a more descriptive and naturalistic methodology to diversifying to embrace other theoretical perspectives, to include symbolic interactionism, critical theory, feminism, and postmodernism. Hammersley and Atkinson (1995) assert that the diversification relates in part to criticisms of the naturalistic approach in that it attempted to understand social phenomena as objects existing independently of the researcher that could be described and even explained in some literal fashion.

Box 2.1

Barclay *et al* (1997) conducted a grounded theory study that explored Australian women's experiences of early motherhood. Data was collected through focus groups and led to the development of six categories: 'realizing'; 'unready'; 'drained'; 'aloneness'; 'loss'; 'working it out'. The core category that integrated the other categories was 'becoming a mother' and this encapsulated the process of change experienced by women. The authors illustrate the connections between the categories in diagrammatic form. The basic social process (Glaser, 1978) of becoming a mother, over a period of time, is explained in narrative form illustrating the links made between categories:

'Realizing' the impact of the child on their lives comes as a shock to mothers. The magnitude of the change they experience and the need to resolve the birth makes it difficult. Women feel 'unready' and are not prepared for the experience of 'becoming a mother'. They feel 'alone' and frequently unsupported by partners, health workers and society as they 'work out' how to become mothers. Women feel 'drained' by physical and emotional fatigue, lack of sleep and the demands of the baby. The experience of new motherhood involves 'losses' which are accompanied by grieving and sometimes resentment. Gains attached to being a mother may take months to be evident but usually compensate women for the losses they experience. Eventually women are able to 'tune in' to their babies as they work out how to 'become mothers' (p. 726).

Symbolic interactionism has had a major influence on the development of ethnography. An ethnography underpinned by a symbolic interactionist theoretical perspective would adopt the view of Hammersley and Atkinson (1995) that people construct their social world through their interpretations of it and their actions are based on their interpretations.

It is also acknowledged that the ethnographer's interpretations are influenced by her/his own culture (Spradley, 1980). As Boyle (1994) notes, ethnography is contextual and reflexive emphasising the importance of context in understanding events and meanings and taking into account the effects of the researcher and the research strategy on findings. It combines both the perspectives of the participant and the researcher.

Box 2.2

Fenwick *et al* (2000) conducted a grounded theory study that explored women's experiences of mothering in an Australian neonatal unit. Data was collected through tape recording interactions between neonatal nurses and mothers. Interviews were conducted with a sample of the mothers and nurses. They found that the verbal exchanges between nurse and mother influenced a woman's confidence, sense of control and her feelings of connection with her infant. They identified two core categories of nursing behaviour, 'facilitative nursing action' and 'inhibitive nursing action' (pp. 199–200). 'Facilitative nursing action' was characterised by nurses 'walking beside the mother', that is, working with the mother, encouraging her and sharing information with her. Secondly, 'women talking' involved the use of positive language that expressed care, support and interest in parents with chatting and use of personal experience being employed in a sensitive way. The third underpinning category involved 'respecting the woman's status as a mother', ie. listening, negotiating, sharing decisions and giving the mother space (p. 199). 'Inhibitive nursing action', on the other hand, involved nurses 'directing the mother and infant' in an authoritative way without listening or negotiating, 'dismissing the woman's rights and skills' and using 'negative language and demeanour'. In addition, the nurses engaged in 'protective care' characterised by a preoccupation with guarding the infant's safety to the detriment of attending to the mother's emotional needs (p. 200). This grounded theory study led to a series of recommendations relating to the importance of the relational aspects of the neonatal nurse-mother encounters.

If the theoretical perspective underpinning ethnography is critical, then the focus will shift to one of ideology, power and transformative action. As Savage (2000: 1401) asserts, critical ethnography attempts to 'restructure the research process in ways that promote the views of those who are silent or marginalised'. Thomas (1993: 3) describes critical ethnography as a:

> *Type of reflection that examines culture, knowledge and action. It expands our horizons for choice and widens our experiential capacity to see, hear and feel. It deepens and sharpens ethical commitments by forcing us to develop and act upon value commitments in the context of political agendas. Critical ethnographers describe, analyze, and open to scrutiny otherwise hidden agendas, power centres, and assumptions that inhibit, repress, and constrain.*

Whichever theoretical perspective underpins ethnography, to achieve a deep level of understanding of a given culture the researcher needs to participate in people's lives over a considerable period of time, to include watching what happens, listening and asking questions (Hammersley and Atkinson, 1995).

In the field of health research, an 'ethnographic approach' rather than a complete ethnography may be adopted to meet the aims of some research projects. The ethnographic approach is topic-orientated in that it focuses upon a specific aspect of activity within a given community (Spradley, 1980).

Two examples of topic-orientated ethnographies are presented (*Boxes 2.3* and *2.4*). These studies illustrate the ways in which the researchers immersed themselves within the cultural settings in order to describe both the culture and the activities and experiences of the social groups involved. Their methods included observation, interviews and field note-taking with each informing the other. In this way, the researchers engaged in 'seeing' as well as 'hearing'. This combination of observing and listening enabled the researchers to contextualise their analyses of cultural themes within a rich description of the cultural setting being studied. Recommendations for cultural change were then made.

Box 2.3

Kirkham and colleagues (Kirkham and Stapleton, 2001a,b; Stapleton *et al*, 2002) combined an ethnographic approach involving observation and interviews with a randomised controlled trial to examine the use of evidence-based leaflets on informed choice in maternity services. The ethnographic research took place in UK maternity units, and included observation of consultations between midwives and service users and interviews with both, combined with comprehensive field note taking. They concluded that while health professionals were positive about the leaflets as a means to facilitate informed choices, competing demands within the clinical environment hindered and undermined their effective use. Time pressures limited opportunities for and depth of discussions between midwives and women. Women's choices were limited by the normative clinical practices with the fear of litigation affecting the way health professionals 'steered' women towards making decisions that maintained the *status quo*. The authors conclude that the culture within which the leaflets were introduced contributed to women engaging in informed compliance rather than making informed choices. This study identifies cultural barriers to implementation of an aspect of best practice, ie. facilitating informed choice within maternity services. Recommendations stemming from the research point to the need for reversal of the considerable cultural inertia that impedes implementation of best practice within maternity services.

Box 2.4

Woodward (2000) adopted a comparative ethnographic study focusing upon the potential contribution of a formal theory of caring upon health care. She observed practices and encounters and conducted interviews with staff in both a palliative nursing setting and a maternity ward. This enabled her to describe key differences between the two cultures. In the palliative care setting, practice was 'other-centred, receptive, responsive and attentive to the patients person and experience' (p. 68). The leadership focused upon team cohesion with regular holding of debriefing meetings in which staff were encouraged to reflect upon care based on theoretical frameworks for caring. Consequently, staff felt motivated, energetic and part of a team. In contrast, practice on the maternity ward was often routinised, task-orientated and sometimes unresponsive to women's needs and the midwives lacked the form of leadership seen in the palliative care setting. Midwives were constrained in developing relationships because of the rapid turnover of women, pressure of work and chronic staff shortages. Their care was often random and non-reflective, without reference to a body of theory underpinning practice. The midwives were left with low levels of motivation and energy. The author recommends that midwifery leaders need to create a culture in which theoretical frameworks are utilised to facilitate critical reflection upon practice that encompasses woman-centred principles and supports the development of a collective vision and way of working for midwives. This requires cultural changes at political, practice and educational levels.

Phenomenological research

Phenomenological research stems from a phenomenological theoretical perspective. However, as stated, the researcher must be clear about which perspective s/he is engaging with, as there are fundamental differences that alter the methodology. For the person considering phenomenological research, Van Manen (1990) provides a useful in-depth text as a starting place. However, the researcher should also read the original texts of the authors whose theoretical perspectives they consider aligning themselves with, so that they may be utilised throughout the research process.

Despite the differences between the branches of phenomenology, it fundamentally differs from other disciplines and their methodologies, as Van Manen (1990: 11) asserts:

> *It does not aim to explicate meanings specific to particular cultures (ethnography), to certain social groups (sociology), to historical periods (history), to mental types (psychology), or to an individual's personal life history (biography).*

Phenomenologists commonly employ in-depth unstructured interviewing with a small number of participants. The analysis is intensive and avoids coding or categorising the data in the ways adopted by, for example grounded theorists. It is not a methodology that may be easily applied to a project that needs the researcher(s) to meet short deadlines with little time for the deep reflection required. The analysis results in the identification of the essence of the studied phenomenon (Van Manen, 1990).

Two examples of phenomenological research are provided (*Boxes 2.5* and *2.6*), both of which make it explicit as to which phenomenological theoretical perspective they draw upon. The first example stems from my own research.

Box 2.5

I adopted a hermeneutic theoretical perspective (Heidegger, 1962) to explore the interpretation of the meaning of women's experiences of breastfeeding, with particular reference to their perceptions related to the adequacy of their breast milk (Dykes and Williams, 1999; Dykes, 2002). The study emphasised the Heideggarian notion that the individual and the world are inextricably linked and therefore pre-understanding cannot be bracketed out to enable the researcher to provide an outside view of the research (Heidegger, 1962; Koch, 1995). Rather, the researcher's socio-political agenda should be made explicit (Burke Draucker, 1999). As Walters (1995) states (p. 798):

According to Heidegger, hermeneutic understanding takes place within a cultural background involving language, personal and bodily practices. This background is always present and can never be made fully explicit. Everyday practical activity receives its meaning from our background of cultural habits.

Women were interviewed at six, twelve and eighteen weeks following birthing. The essence of the breastfeeding experience was illustrated through the metaphor 'falling by the wayside' (Dykes and Williams, 1999). This reflected the challenges that women experienced on their breastfeeding journey and the differences between expectations and their realities. Women tended to adopt mechanistic, dualistic and reductionist assumptions regarding breastfeeding. They endeavoured to quantify and visualise their breast milk and monitor 'output' to the baby through weighing and related techniques. They powerfully highlighted their unmet needs for social support, nurturing and replenishment. Recommendations were made to improve social and health professional support for breastfeeding women, particularly within communities where breastfeeding is a marginal activity and associated social support networks are largely inadequate.

Feminist standpoint research

Feminist standpoint research stems from a feminist theoretical perspective. It may merge with another methodology, so that the research could be referred to as, for example, a feminist ethnography or feminist action research. Feminist standpoint research may draw upon a wide range of qualitative methods, for example, interviewing, focus groups and observation. Some feminists utilise quantitative methodologies, if felt to be appropriate, to answer specific questions in specific ways (Oakley, 1992, 2000).

Feminist methodology is concerned with the place of women throughout the research process. This is summarised by Carter (1995: 12) who states:

Feminist approaches necessitate understanding women's experiences in relation to patriarchal social relations. More fundamental than the questions asked by the researcher are the intentions behind the research, the ways in which responses are understood and the theoretical perspectives which frame the discussion.

Box 2.6

The phenomenological research of Halldorsdottir (1996) focused upon the essential structure of caring and uncaring encounters with midwives and nurses, from the clients' perspectives within a range of health care settings in Iceland (Halldorsdottir, 1991; Halldorsdottir and Karlsdottir, 1996a,b; Halldorsdottir, 1996). The phenomenological methodology utilised for this study was inspired by Ricoeur (1990) and Anderson (1991). This provided a 'unique blend of description, interpretation and construction' (Halldorsdottir and Karlsdottir, 1996a, p. 137). The essence of the experience of caring and uncaring encounters was illustrated through the metaphors, of 'the bridge' and 'the wall' with the former leading to 'empowerment' and the latter to 'discouragement' (Halldorsdottir, 1996, p. 30). The 'bridge' symbolised a trusting, connected, caring relationship based on respect and open forms of communication and seeing the person being cared for in her/his own inner and outer contexts, resulting in the client feeling empowered. In contrast, the 'wall' represented poor communication, 'detachment' and 'lack of a caring' connection (Halldorsdottir 1996, p. 5). More specifically the nurse appeared to be 'disinterested', 'insensitive' and 'cold/business-like' (p. 36). A sense of mutual avoidance developed with the 'nurse being perceived as unwilling or unable to connect with the patient' (p. 32). This form of encounter created a lack of trust and the client experienced discouragement, a sense of aloneness, insecurity and anxiety, lowering of confidence, decreased sense of being in control and sometimes a sense of failure. Midwifery and nursing practice issues stemming from the findings were subsequently highlighted.

There are three strongly identifiable characteristics within qualitative feminist standpoint methodologies, although they are not unique to feminism. Firstly, reflexivity is considered to be crucial, as illustrated throughout the edited works of Ribbens and Edwards (1998). As Mauthner and Doucet (1998: 127) assert, being reflexive about data analysis involves:

Locating ourselves socially in relation to our respondent; attending to our emotional responses to this person and examining how we make theoretical interpretations of the respondent's narrative.

To achieve this a:

Profound level of self-awareness is required to begin to capture the perspectives through which we view the world; and it is not easy to grasp the 'unconscious' filters through which we experience the world.

Mauthner and Doucet, 1998: 122

The other characteristics of feminist methodologies include attention to a transformative and emancipatory potential and the notion of inter-subjectivity. Inter-subjectivity relates to acknowledgement of the reciprocal nature of the encounter with meaning being constructed by the researcher and participants (Burman, 1992; Stanley and Wise, 1993; Standing, 1998).

Two examples of feminist standpoint research are provided (*Boxes 2.7* and *2.8*). A feminist theoretical perspective informed both studies, with the authors conducting and interpreting their research in a way that identified the dilemmas and struggles for women in situations in which patriarchal systems place constraints upon women.

Box 2.7

Carter (1995) conducted feminist standpoint research to elicit the retrospective experiences of breastfeeding for a cohort of women who had their babies between 1920 and 1980. Her interviews revealed that for working class women there were clear conditions that precluded against prolonged and exclusive breastfeeding. These included unhealthy working conditions that were hazardous, time-consuming and exhausting. Housing was often cramped with more than one generation co-existing. Breastfeeding became a symbol of poverty associated with tough living conditions, large families, exhaustion, poverty, discomfort, embarrassment and restriction. Given the relentless demands upon women, Carter (1995) argues that bottle feeding appeared to have given them a sense of control over their lives. It also enabled them to resist the exhortations to self-monitor their bodies and control aspects of their lives that were considered to affect their milk. A growing antipathy towards breastfeeding was compounded by authoritarianism combined with insufficient support in hospital and inadequate family support at home (Carter, 1995).

Box 2.8

Edwards (2000, 2001) conducted a series of in-depth interviews with women who planned to have home births in Scotland. Through in-depth analysis of women's experiences she highlighted the dominance of the techno-medical model of birth and the lack of robust alternatives. This limited the women's and midwives' abilities to construct their own birthing knowledge and practices and hindered the forming of trusting, supportive relationships between mothers and midwives. Edwards (2000: 80) illustrates the ways in which women and midwives attempt to function in an unsupportive, hierarchical structure:

In the same way that midwives felt unable to assert themselves for fear of reprisal, many women in this study felt unable to assert their needs for fear of causing further tensions in fragile relationships on which they would depend at a time of vulnerability.

Conclusion

It is clear that each theoretical perspective and methodology has undergone a complex 'journey' with changing and differing views being expressed along the way. To add to the complexity, researchers are increasingly merging theoretical perspectives and methodologies, resulting in hybrid approaches to research. The controversies and debates are likely to continue and, as this happens, adaptation, attenuation, hybridisation and expansion will continue to occur. Given these complexities, the descriptions presented constitute an overview only, however, the references provide a useful resource for further reading.

The examples of research, presented above, cover a range of issues relating to women's experiences of pregnancy, labour and birth, early motherhood and breastfeeding. They also highlight the influence of health system cultures upon women's experiences and on health staff supporting them. They illuminate ways in which women may experience supportive and unsupportive encounters within health systems and wider community settings. The examples illustrate the ways in which qualitative studies vary depending upon the theoretical perspectives and methodologies employed, but that synergies may be seen when the findings are viewed collectively. Becoming aware of the resonance between study findings is one of the exciting aspects of reading qualitative research conducted from different perspectives within a range of settings and contexts.

References

Aamodt A (1991) Ethnography and epistemology: generating nursing knowledge. In: Morse J, ed. *Qualitative Nursing Research: A Contemporary Dialogue*. Sage, London: 40–53

Anderson J (1991) The phenomenological perspective. In: Morse J, ed. *Qualitative Nursing Research: A Contemporary Dialogue*. Sage, London: 25–38

Barclay L (1997) Becoming a mother — an analysis of women's experience of early motherhood. *J Adv Nurs* **25**: 719–28

Berger P, Luckmann T (1967) *The Social Construction of Reality: A Treatise in the Sociology of Knowledge*. Penguin books, Harmondsworth

Blumer H (1969) *Symbolic Interactionism: Perspective and Method*. Prentice Hall, Englewood Cliffs

Boyle J (1994) Styles of ethnography. In: Morse J, ed. *Critical Issues in Qualitative Research Methods*. Sage, London: 158–9

Burke Draucker C (1999) The critique of Heideggarian hermeneutical nursing research. *J Adv Nurs* **30**(2): 360–73

Burman E (1992) Feminism and discourse in developmental psychology: power, subjectivity and interpretation. *Feminism and Psychology* **2**(1): 45–60

Carter J (1995) *Feminism, Breasts and Breastfeeding*. Macmillan Press, London

Crotty M (1998) *The Foundations of Social Research: Meaning and Perspective in the Research Process*. Sage Publications, London

Davis-Floyd R, St John G (1998) *From Doctor to Healer — The Transformative Journey*. Rutgers University Press, London

Deery R, Kirkham M (2000) Moving from hierarchy to collaboration. The birth of an action research project. *Practis Midwife* **3**(80): 25–8

Denzin N, Lincoln Y (1994) Major paradigms and perspectives. In: Denzin N, Lincoln Y, eds. *Handbook of Qualitative Research*. Sage Publications, London: 99–104

Dykes F, Williams C (1999) 'Falling by the Wayside' A phenomenological exploration of perceived breast milk inadequacy in lactating women. *Midwif* **15**: 232–46

Dykes F (2002) Western marketing and medicine — construction of an insufficient milk syndrome. *Health Care for Women International* **23**(5): 492–502

Edwards N (2000) Women planning home births: their views on their relationships with midwives. In Kirkham M, ed. *The Midwife-Mother Relationship*. Macmillan Press, London: 55–91

Edwards N (2001) *Women's experiences of planning home births in Scotland — Birthing Autonomy*. Unpublished PhD thesis, University of Sheffield, UK

Fenwick J, Barclay L, Schmied V (2000) Interactions in neonatal nurseries: women's perceptions of nurses and nursing. *J Neonatal Nurs* **6**(6): 197–203

Fox NJ (1993) *Postmodernism, Sociology and Health*. Open University Press, Buckingham

Gadamer HG (1976) *Philosophical Hermeneutics*. University of California Press, Berkeley

Glaser BG, Strauss AL (1967) *The Discovery of Grounded Theory: Strategies for Qualitative Research*. Aldine, Chicago

Glaser BG (1978) *Theoretical Sensitivity*. Sociology Press, Mill Valley, California

Goffman E (1959) *The Presentation of Self in Everyday Life*. Penguin, Harmondsworth

Guba E, Lincoln Y (1994) Competing paradigms in qualitative research. In: Denzin N, Lincoln Y, eds. *Handbook of Qualitative Research*. Sage Publications, London: 105–117

Habermas J (1972) *Knowledge and Human Interests*. Heinemann, London

Halldorsdottir S (1991) Five basic modes of being with another. In: Gaut DA, Leininger MM, eds. *Caring: The Compassionate Healer*. National League for Nursing, New York: 37–49

Halldorsdottir S (1996) *Caring and Uncaring Encounters in Nursing and Health Care — Developing a Theory*. PhD by publication, Linkoping University, Sweden.

Halldorsdottir S, Karlsdottir SI (1996a) Empowerment or discouragement: Women's experiences of caring and uncaring encounters during childbirth. *Health Care for Women International* **17**(4): 135–52

Halldorsdottir S, Karlsdottir SI (1996b) Journeying through labour and delivery: perceptions of women who have given birth. *Midwif* **12**: 48–61

Hammersley M, Atkinson P (1995) *Ethnography: Principles in Practice*. 2nd edn. Routledge, London

Heidegger M (1962) *Being and Time*. Basil Blackwell, Oxford

Helman C (1994) *Culture, Health and Illness*. 3rd edn. Butterworth-Heinemann, Oxford

Humm M (1992) *Feminisms. A Reader*. Harvester Wheatsheaf, Hertfordshire

Husserl E (1931) *Ideas: General Introduction to Pure Phenomenology*. George Allen and Unwin, London

Husserl E (1970) *The Crisis of European Sciences and Transcendental Phenomenology: An Introduction to Phenomenological Philosophy*. North Western University Press, Evanston

Husserl E (1973) *The Idea of Phenomenology*. Martinus Nijhoff, The Hague

Kendall G, Wickham G (1999) *Using Foucault's Methods*. Sage Publications, London

Kincheloe JL, McClaren PL (1994) Rethinking critical theory and qualitative research. In: Denzin NK, Lincoln YS, eds. *Handbook of Qualitative Research*. Sage publications, London: 138–57

Kirkham M, Stapleton H, eds (2001a) *Informed Choice in Maternity Care: An Evaluation of Evidence Based Leaflets*. NHS Centre for Reviews and Dissemination, University of York, York

Kirkham M, Stapleton H (2001b) The ethnographic study. In: Kirkham M, Stapleton H, eds. *Informed Choice in Maternity Care: An Evaluation of Evidence Based Leaflets*. NHS Centre for Reviews and Dissemination, University of York, York: 13–22

Koch T (1995) Interpretive approaches in nursing research: the influence of Husserl and Heidegger. *J Adv Nurs* **21**: 827–36

Kuhn TS (1970) *The Structure of Scientific Revolutions*. Chicago University Press, Chicago

Latour B (1987) *Science in Action: How to Follow Engineers in Society*. Open University Press, Milton Keynes

Mason J (1996) *Qualitative Researching*. Sage Publications, London

Mauthner M, Doucet A (1998) Analysing maternal and domestic discourses. In: Ribbens J, Edwards R, eds (1998) *Feminist Dilemmas in Qualitative Research*. Sage Publications, London: 39–57

Mead GH (1934) *Mind, Self and Society*. University of Chicago Press, Chicago

Murphy E, Dingwall R, Greatbatch D, Parker S and Watson P (1998) Qualitative research methods in health technology assessment: a review of the literature. *Health Technol Assess* **2**(16). Online at: www.hta.nhsweb.nhs.uk\fullmono\mon216.pdf

Oakley A (1992) *Social Support and Motherhood*. Basil Blackwell, Oxford

Oakley A (2000) *Experiments in Knowing: Gender and Method in the Social Sciences*. Polity Press, Cambridge

Reason P (1994) *Participation in Human Inquiry*. Sage publications, London

Ribbens J, Edwards R, eds (1998) *Feminist Dilemmas in Qualitative Research*. Sage Publications, London

Ricoeur P (1990) *Hermeneutics and the Human Sciences: Essays on and Interpretation*. Cambridge University Press, Cambridge

Rogan F, Schmied V, Barclay L, Everitt L, Wyllie A (1997) 'Becoming a mother' — developing a new theory of early motherhood. *J Adv Nurs* **25**: 877–85

Savage J (2000) Ethnography and health care. *Br Med J* **321**: 1400–02

Shildrick M (1997) *Leaky Bodies and Boundaries: Feminism, postmodernism and (bio)ethics*. Routledge, London

Spradley (1980) *Participant Observation*. Holt, Rinehart and Winston, USA

Stapleton H, Kirkham M, Thomas G (2002) Qualitative study of evidence based leaflets in maternity care. *Br Med J* **324**: 1–6

Standing K (1998) Writing the voices of the less powerful. In: Ribbens J, Edwards R, eds. *Feminist Dilemmas in Qualitative Research*. Sage Publications, London: 24–38

Stanley L, Wise S (1993) *Breaking Out Again: Feminist Ontology and Epistemology*. Routledge, London

Strauss A, Corbin J (1990) *Basics of Qualitative Research. Grounded theory procedures and techniques*. Sage, London

Thomas J (1993) *Doing Critical Ethnography. Qualitative Researchs Methods*. Vol. 26, Sage, London

Tong RP (1998) *Feminist Thought: A More Comprehensive Introduction*. Westview Press, Oxford

Turner BS (1987) *Medical Power and Social Knowledge*. Sage, London

Turner BS (1992) *Regulating Bodies: Essays in Medical Sociology*. Routledge, London

Van Manen M (1990) *Researching Lived Experience, Human Science for an Action Sensitive Pedagogy.* State University of New York Press, New York

Walters AJ (1995) The phenomenological movement: implications for nursing research. *J Adv Nurs* **22**: 791–99

Woodward V (2000) Caring for women: the potential contribution of formal theory to midwifery practice. *Midwif* **16**: 68–75

Chapter 3

What are the ethical considerations?

Donal Manning

> *Equals be treated equally, and unequals unequally in*
> *proportion to the relevant inequalities.*
>
> Aristotle 384 BC–322 BC

Introduction

Some researchers argue that ethical issues in qualitative social science research differ from those in quantitative biomedical research, and thus that the former is not best served by the conventional 'biomedical' approach to research ethics review (Murphy *et al*, 1998). I hope to show, however, that in qualitative research in health care, while there may be differences in emphasis from quantitative research, the ethical issues in both types of research are essentially the same. In this chapter, I will review briefly the main ethical theories and principles informing healthcare research, and the historical background to research ethics. I will then discuss ethical issues in qualitative research, and finally offer advice on applying for ethics committee approval. Unless otherwise specified, by research I mean research in health care.

Healthcare ethics — an overview

Consequentialism and deontological theories have dominated biomedical ethics in the past fifty years. Consequentialist theories hold that the foreseeable consequences of a given action are the only aspects of the action that matter morally (Hope *et al*, 2003). Utilitarianism, the best known consequentialist theory, holds that the moral value of an action is measured in terms of the net overall happiness that is produced by doing that action. At first glance, consequentialism is intuitively attractive. It makes sense to act so as to produce more good than harm. Much healthcare practice may appear to be guided by utilitarian considerations, such as prescribing cancer chemotherapy if the side-effects are calculated to be outweighed by improved life expectancy or quality of life, and immunisation programmes, where the adverse effects (and the overriding of individual choice) are calculated to be outweighed by the communal benefits.

However, consequentialism suffers from significant defects (Hope *et al*, 2003: 5). It is impersonal, calculating communal benefit possibly at the expense of individual, personal, considerations. It depends crucially on calculation of benefits and harms, but what counts as these is difficult to settle, and measuring health goods and harms is difficult. This is a particular problem in research, when there is inherent uncertainty regarding outcomes, good or bad. There may also be problems with just distribution of goods, and taken literally, consequentialism could justify immoral practice. For example, if benefit-harm analysis suggested that providing a health intervention to the rich produced greater utility than offering it to the poor, the strict consequentialist would require us to offer the intervention to the better off. Powerful intuitions would suggest that helping the rich and depriving the poor is immoral, regardless of the consequences. In the research context, consequentialism could theoretically justify dispensing with informed consent if this increased recruitment to a study that might produce substantial communal benefit.

Deontological (duty-based) theory in a sense takes the opposite view to consequentialism. It holds that aspects of an action, other than its consequences, such as the motives, intentions and duties of the agent, matter morally (Hope *et al*, 2003: 6). Persons should do the right thing, according to their duties and responsibilities, consequences notwithstanding. Duties are often expressed in negative terms (constraints), such as the duty not to lie, or the duty not to violate an individual's rights. Kant, considered to be the father of deontology, held that universal moral rules, derived rationally, should be followed unconditionally. Deontological theory accords great moral value to autonomy and respect for persons. One formulation of Kant's unconditional (categorical) imperative states that moral agents should not be treated solely as means, but also as ends in themselves (Hope *et al*, 2003: 7). Obvious medical applications of this constraint prohibit health professionals from deceiving or coercing patients into undergoing treatment or taking part in research.

Like consequentialism, deontology has its problems. Of course the consequences of our actions matter morally, and a theory that demanded absolute adherence to abstract rules, with no regard to consequences, would not be viable. Autonomy can be overridden justifiably if respecting it might have extreme consequences for the community. Thus, in the case of serious communicable disease, liberty and confidentiality can be waived, through quarantine and notification, in the communal interest. Autonomy is also not the overriding moral consideration for individuals with limited or no autonomy, such as infants, young children and the mentally ill. For these individuals, protecting them from harm and promoting their best interests are the main moral considerations, both in clinical care and research. In research, the injunction, expressed in the Nuremberg code (Shuster, 1997: 1436), that the consent of the participant is absolutely essential, if taken literally, would disqualify all research on neonates, young children, and those with severe mental illness and dementia. Yet the consequences of this approach would be unacceptable, and failure to conduct research, for example in neonatal intensive care and Alzheimer's disease, would discriminate against the relevant subjects.

As we have seen, neither of the great moral theories can capture fully the complexity of healthcare ethics. Either theory, if followed rigidly, could produce moral guidance that is counterintuitive. Another approach, based on applying moral principles, rather than comprehensive theories, to bioethical problems, has been formulated by Beauchamp and Childress (2001), and promoted in Britain by Gillon (1986). They outline four principles:

i **Beneficence** stresses the obligation to do good to others. It emphasises high standards of professional practice, for example commitment to continuing professional education and to practice according to the best available evidence.

ii **Non-maleficence** prohibits doing harm. It is not absolute — if so, it would prohibit any medical intervention that had potential adverse effects. Also, it is not simply the mirror image of beneficence, since the principles have different scope. Thus, the obligation not to harm others is arguably universal, whereas the obligation of beneficence cannot be so wide, but is directly to specific persons, such as a health professional's patients.

Many health care interventions involve weighing beneficence and non-maleficence, such as estimating risk-benefit analysis in cancer chemotherapy, or in immunisation programmes, and these two principles have obvious application to consequentialist theory. They are clearly relevant to weighing the risks and benefits of research.

iii **Respect for autonomy** underpins the right of autonomous agents to self-determination. In health care, it demands that professionals respect the right of competent patients to choose between alternative treatments, and it is fundamental to informed consent. It also underpins rights to privacy and confidentiality, and is clearly applicable therefore to research ethics. Part of the justification of respect for autonomy is that a competent person, not her doctor, is the best judge of what counts as good or bad outcomes for her. However, the principle goes further than this, and requires us to respect patient choice even if this might lead to adverse consequences, such as the refusal by a Jehovah's Witness of life-saving blood transfusion. The principle thus has clear deontologic force (though Mill, 1991, claimed that respecting autonomy and human flourishing was part of his utilitarian conception of the good).

iv **Justice**, to paraphrase Aristotle, holds that 'equals be treated equally, and unequals unequally in proportion to the relevant inequalities' (Gillon, 1986: 87–88). Thus, people with equivalent needs, rights or deserts should be treated similarly. The clearest applications in health care are in distribution of scarce resources. There is no universal agreement on what the morally relevant criteria for acting justly are: should healthcare goods be distributed according to need, merit, or utility? In research ethics, justice demands that the benefits and burdens of research be shared fairly by different groups in the community.

The 'four principles' approach has been very influential in healthcare ethics, and it provides a useful framework for appraising bioethical problems. Like the major theories, it has been criticised for being abstract and ignoring context and the individual dimension in ethical dilemmas, and it has been derided for offering a 'cookbook' approach to ethical problem-solving. It has also been criticised for promoting a middle-class, Western perspective in bioethics. In particular, the great value placed on autonomy has been charged with promoting a self-centred, individualistic ethic at the expense of a more caring, communitarian approach.

These accounts of consequentialism, deontology and principlism are necessarily simplistic, and much more sophisticated versions have been developed which to some extent address many of the above criticisms. While other theoretical approaches have attracted increasing attention recently, such as virtue theory, and feminist, care-based, pragmatic and narrative ethics, the two classical ethical theories still hold centre stage. Although simplified, these descriptions of consequentialism and deontology offer a metaphor for the inherent tension in research, between the consequentialist imperative to discover knowledge and the deontological requirement to respect participants. In principlist terms, the tension is between beneficence and respect for autonomy. The history of biomedical research and, indeed, of much qualitative research, reflects these tensions.

The historical background to research ethics

Ethical codes of practice governing research, such as the Nuremberg Code (Shuster, 1997) and the Declaration of Helsinki (World Medical Association, 2000), evolved in response to the scandals of Nazi 'medical' experimentation and the post-war recognition in both Britain and the United States that research was being conducted, often on vulnerable people, without any attempts to gain their consent (Beecher, 1966; Papworth, 1967). Concern about these abuses reached a crescendo with the uncovering of the Tuskegee scandal, in which poor black American men with syphilis were deceived into partaking in a 'study' of the natural history of untreated syphilis (Caplan, 1992). This study, conducted after penicillin had been recognised as an effective treatment for the disease, continued unchecked for about forty years until 1972. In response to the outrage caused by the discovery of this scandal, the US Congress set up the infrastructure for institutional review board (the American equivalent of our research ethics committees) approval of research (Caplan, 1992). In Britain, the regulation of research has developed along similar lines, culminating in the recent publication of the research governance framework for health and social care (Department of Health, 2001a).

Rothman (1987) argues that the abuses cited in Beecher's famous article reflected a post-war utilitarian ethic, which held that the supposed benefits of research outweighed the harms caused by ignoring individual rights. Societal trends in the past fifty years have rejected this ethic in favour of increasing respect for autonomy and rights, and these trends are reflected in codes of ethical practice, the writings of bioethicists and the attitudes of research ethics committees. All place a high premium on seeking informed consent. The Nuremberg Code states that the consent of the individual to take part in research is absolutely essential, and the Declaration of Helsinki states that the benefits to society of conducting research must not take precedence over the well-being and rights of participants.

Interestingly, the history of social sciences research shows some parallels to the utilitarianism of early biomedical research, in which the ends of uncovering new knowledge were justified by what would now be considered unethical means. Rosenhan (1973), for example, published the experiences of a group of observers who fabricated symptoms of schizophrenia and were admitted to psychiatric hospitals. Once admitted, they stopped fabricating and resumed 'normal' behaviour. Nonetheless, their behaviour was consistently interpreted by the staff as pathological and many were labelled, even after discharge, as being schizophrenics in remission. While this famous paper may have uncovered valuable insights into the medicalisation of behaviour and of psychiatric practice, nowadays the gross deception committed would not be considered justifiable as a means to the end of obtaining this information.

Punch (1998) has provided many other examples of qualitative research that involved covert observation or frank deceit, which underline the tension between the imperatives to discover new information, and to do so ethically. Since the Department of Health's research governance framework clearly and repeatedly places research in health and social care together in outlining good research practice, qualitative researchers in health care have no option but to adhere to research practice that has largely been informed by the biomedical model.

Ethical issues in qualitative research

Methodological issues

The methodological quality of a proposal is a fundamental ethical issue. Bad science is unethical. It is wrong to prevail upon people to undertake the commitments and possible risks of partaking in research, which is so poorly designed that it cannot generate valid and interpretable knowledge. Society, too, may be harmed if health professionals, legislators and administrators act upon misleading information generated by such research. Health professionals, familiar with the predictability, objectivity and statistical rigour of quantitative research, often struggle to assess qualitative research, with its emphasis on small numbers, exploration of subjective experience and unpredictable and unfolding nature (Cribb, 2003).

Nonetheless, there are standards that can help guide the conduct and evaluation of qualitative research. The two broad criteria for assessing research quality are **validity** and **relevance** (Mays and Pope, 2000). Validity can be promoted by attention to the aspects of qualitative research that are covered in greater detail in other chapters, including triangulation, respondent validation and reflexivity (Mays and Pope, 2000).

The relevance of a qualitative study is judged by the extent to which the findings add to current knowledge, and by the confidence with which they are regarded (Mays and Pope, 2000). These are obviously related to validity. While qualitative research data are not generalisable in the same numerical sense as quantitative research, if the data are valid and relevant, they may be applicable to similar groups or persons, they may add to theory, and may be 'conceptually' generalisable (Green, 1999). Reliability in collecting the data, selecting extracts for illustration, and in publishing the findings are not just methodological, but also ethical issues.

Harm

Qualitative research demands considerable expertise, and appropriate education and training of investigators is important. If the researcher is inexperienced or unskilled, participants may be harmed. While research ethics review has been informed by awareness that biomedical research can put participants at significant harm, qualitative research has sometimes been assumed to be risk-free. Neither generalisation is fully correct. There is increasing evidence that participation in well-reviewed, conducted and monitored biomedical research carries an inclusion benefit, not only for subjects receiving the treatment under investigation, but also for those receiving standard treatment (Chalmers and Lindley, 2001: 270). Also, qualitative research can cause harm, and since benefit to individual participants cannot be assumed, weighing the harm-benefit ratio should focus almost exclusively on potential harms.

Ironically, the more in depth the probing in qualitative research, the greater is the potential for harm (Cribb, 2003: 44–45). Qualitative research typically involves exploring personal experience in depth and this process, when applied to people's experience of illness and treatment, can evoke strong emotional responses and distress. This is unsurprising when researching traumatic experiences, such as postnatal depression and termination of pregnancy, but it may apply to almost any exploration of persons' experience of illness. Also, the potential for harm is unpredictable — some participants may find involvement in interviews or focus groups therapeutic, while some may be traumatised. Researchers must be prepared to deal with the distress which may be elicited in these settings, and to have arrangements in place to offer expert support for this eventuality (Cribb, 2003: 45).

Participants may also be harmed if there is a blurring of the distinction between professional and investigator roles. If the research involves in depth exploration of sensitive personal issues, participants may feel let down or betrayed when the investigator, whom they may have come to see as a confidante or friend, withdraws when the research is finished. In research, assessing the quality of, or access to, a given treatment, there is the added potential risk of unduly raising participants' expectations.

Further potential for harm arises from possible breach of confidentiality, and I will discuss this below.

Consent

Informed consent demands reasonable communication of relevant information, the ability of the recipient to understand this information, and the freedom to decide whether or not to take part (Beauchamp and Childress, 2001). The evolving nature of qualitative research projects poses a challenge to communication of information. Important issues may only emerge as the research develops, so giving a full account of the nature of the study at the outset may be impossible (Murphy *et al*, 1998). To counter this, it has been suggested that consent should be a 'process', not a one-off signing of a form (Ramcharan and Cutcliffe, 2001). Participants should be kept informed about the evolution of the project, and be at liberty to withdraw at any stage.

Given the theoretical complexity of qualitative research, and its relative unfamiliarity to both lay people and health professionals, it is important to establish the competence of individuals to understand what participating in the study might entail for them. The onus is on the investigator to provide clear written and verbal information on the nature and purpose of the study. This should be tailored to the needs of specific participant groups, such as competent adults, minors, and people with learning difficulties. Arrangements may be needed for translation of study documentation, particularly the information leaflet and consent form, and interpretation, to facilitate inclusion of participants from ethnic minorities.

Voluntariness is a particular issue in research conducted by a professional who is also providing clinical care to the participant. Patients should not feel obliged to participate by debt of gratitude to their clinician, or through fear that their care may be compromised if they refuse. Treading the line between seeking voluntary consent and subtle coercion can be difficult for researchers, who are understandably keen to recruit participants, but who must present the request to participate in as neutral a manner as possible.

Conducting observational research in clinical areas, such as inpatient wards and intensive care units, poses particular challenges to seeking informed consent (Murphy *et al*, 1998). Such research can involve close observation, over extended periods, of different health professionals, patients and other lay people. Who should consent to being observed? If a departmental head agrees to the research taking place, can subordinate professionals refuse? If the research is in teamwork and clinical care, is the consent of patients needed? What is the difference between a public setting, where observation is a normal social activity, and a private one, where consent and confidentiality must be respected (Murphy *et al*, 1998; Punch, 1998)? In research of this nature, seeking the consent of all potential subjects may be impractical. There is also the theoretical concern that awareness of being observed might influence the behaviour of individuals, thus invalidating the research. There are no easy or universally agreed solutions to these difficulties, and each situation must be judged on its merits. While some observational research might be justifiable without the explicit consent of all those being observed, what is clear is that covert research, involving deception or disguise, is rarely, if ever, acceptable in the healthcare setting (Murphy *et al*, 1998).

Confidentiality

Confidentiality may be more difficult to protect in qualitative than in quantitative research (Murphy *et al*, 1998). In quantitative research there is often safety in numbers, whereas qualitative research is typically conducted on a smaller scale, and so there is greater potential for individuals or groups to be identifiable. As Punch (1998) has pointed out, most academic units conduct research in their surrounding neighbourhood, and local research, for example, in teenage abortion, may identify a defined group of participants.

Qualitative researchers may obtain sensitive personal information during their work, participants may drop their guard and disclose more than may be in their best interests, and some such information might be of interest to the courts or police (Murphy *et al*, 1998). Investigators have a substantial moral obligation to protect the identity of participants. On the other hand, if the investigator receives information that might suggest that an individual is at risk of serious harm, for example, child sexual abuse, there may be a moral, and legal, obligation to breach confidentiality.

In contrast to quantitative research, in qualitative research the greatest risks to confidentiality occur during publication and dissemination of the findings, not during the research itself (Murphy *et al*, 1998: 153). Groups as well as individuals may be at risk from stigmatisation or victim-blaming. The use of pseudonyms and related methods may be necessary, and when including verbatim transcripts in the published report, the investigator should take care to ensure that this does not give clues to the identity of the narrator.

Participants, no less than investigators, must be reminded of their obligations to confidentiality, to avoid hearsay, and to respect the privacy of personal information which might be divulged, for example in focus groups, or in observational research in a clinical area.

Writing up and disseminating the research findings

Integrity is fundamental to qualitative research, which by its nature is subjective, and there is substantial scope for misinterpretation, and for being selective in presenting the findings. Quantitative research can provide safeguards with its onus on inclusion and exclusion criteria, allowing for confounding factors, rigorous statistical analysis, data monitoring committees and stopping rules. As outlined above, there are standards of rigour for qualitative research, but much more depends on the investigator in terms of rigour of analysis, reflexivity and honesty in writing up the research.

All too often in qualitative research, the findings are not shared sufficiently widely, but are just used towards the end of obtaining a degree. While they may not be as generalisable as the findings of quantitative research, the findings may offer theoretical or empirical suggestions that may inform practice and research more widely than the narrow context of the initial study. Dissemination of good quality research findings is an ethical imperative.

In summary, while there are differences in emphasis between the two types of research, the principles of ethically sound research are common to both quantitative and qualitative research. Poor quality research is unethical, informed consent is fundamental, participants must be protected from harm, their confidentiality and privacy must be respected, and the investigator must be honest in writing up the findings, which should usually be disseminated.

Applying for research ethics committee approval

Ethics committees have the dual remit of protecting the dignity and rights of participants, and of facilitating ethically sound research. Their relationship with researchers is sometimes adversarial, implying a tension between these responsibilities. This should not necessarily be the case — ethical research should by definition protect the dignity and rights of participants. If investigators acknowledged the two responsibilities facing committees, and that they should be complementary, they could save themselves much grief (and delay) in seeking ethical approval.

Preparing a project for ethical review involves attending to the ethical issues that I have outlined above, and I will therefore use broadly the same headings in offering suggestions to help the researcher in this.

Methodological issues

Ethics committee members are often less familiar with qualitative than with quantitative research methodology. They may struggle with theoretical issues, the small numbers of proposed participants, the inherent subjectivity, the limited generalisability of the findings, the lack of an initial hypothesis and the notion of emergent research unfolding unpredictably. Until recently, not all British committees have had members with expertise in qualitative research, although the governance arrangements for research ethics committees recommend that nowadays they should (Department of Health, 2001b). Experienced researchers often express frustration when a committee appears not to understand the nature of, and justification for, their application. While this frustration is understandable, ethics committees are a useful barometer of both professional and lay understanding. If a group of relatively well educated and interested adults is unable to grasp the nature and purpose of a proposed research project, an average group of patients, who may be acutely or chronically ill and feeling vulnerable is even less likely to do so. The investigators are responsible for making the study reasonably understandable.

Providing an independent critique of the study would go a long way toward facilitating ethical review, and might lead to approval of the application at the first attempt. This is a difficult issue, and the research governance framework does not take a rigid line, suggesting that for student projects an internal critique may suffice (Department of Health, 2001b). In quantitative research, the request for external critiques is routinely ignored by pharmaceutical companies, and so committees find it difficult to insist on receiving critiques of other projects. Funding from one of the major research funding bodies is reasonably reassuring evidence of the scientific merit of a proposed study, but most inexperienced researchers will not be in such a fortunate position. Letters of commendation from supervisors or academic boards may imply methodological endorsement of a proposal, but if there are difficult methodological issues or other substantial ethical concerns, an independent critique would be helpful.

How should investigators obtain independent review of their proposed study? Academics are busy people, and perhaps cannot reasonably be expected to offer their services free. Perhaps academic departments could work together to offer reciprocal, though independent, review. This would be in the interests of investigators, because if the ethics committee have significant doubts about methodological issues, approval may be delayed while the committee defers, or commissions its own review.

While some researchers instinctively dislike a checklist approach to ethical review, it can offer a useful framework for both investigators and ethics committee members. Mays and Pope (2000) suggest a checklist for assessing study quality, with headings including relevance of the project, clarity of the research question, appropriateness of the study design, attention to context, and evidence of reflexivity. This list is not exhaustive, and all headings may not be appropriate for all submissions, but it could provide a useful benchmark for submitting and assessing qualitative research projects.

The application should give a clear account of the nature and purpose of the proposal. Why is the topic important? What is already known about it? What will this study add? How will it be conducted? This information should be outlined at the start of the protocol. All too often, the study background appears to be a transcription of chapter 1 of the investigator's Master's dissertation. Ethics committees prefer much more concise and simple accounts of the study background. Inexperienced investigators tend to use long words and sentences — avoid jargon about grounded theory, hermeneutics and paradigms. Stick to plain English. An ability to explain clearly the study background and outline is reassuring evidence that the investigator herself understands it.

The proposal should describe the experience of the investigator in qualitative research methodology, or what training will be undertaken by inexperienced researchers before embarking on the study. If sensitive topics are to be explored, or if participants are likely to be particularly vulnerable, it should say what arrangements are in place to offer professional support in the event of participants becoming very distressed.

Consent

The participant information leaflet should take into account the three components of informed consent: information sharing; promoting participant understanding; and assurance on voluntariness. As such, it is one of the documents to which ethics committees devote most attention. Providing written information gives no guarantee of adequate verbal communication, no more than a signed form is evidence of informed consent, but if care is not devoted to the information leaflet, committees may surmise that verbal communication between investigator and potential participant will be no better.

The leaflet should state clearly that the proposed study is research, and not give the impression that it is an extension of therapeutic care. It should describe clearly the rationale for doing the study, and what participation would involve. It is important for investigators to be honest. If the study is about postnatal depression, investigators should say so, and avoid euphemisms such as 'exploring women's feelings after delivery'.

If the emergent and unpredictable nature of the research is acknowledged openly, committees will understand that full disclosure of all possible eventualities cannot be given at the outset. It is best to acknowledge uncertainty. In fact, in this regard, qualitative research does not differ greatly from quantitative research. Uncertainty is an inherent aspect of research. Even in the classic randomised controlled trial, the study outcome cannot always be predicted — if it could, arguably the study would be unethical. Consent as a process, to be revisited as the study evolves, if appropriate, should be outlined.

Investigators should be frank about what commitment the participant undertakes by consenting, including the anticipated number and length of interviews. Committees are sceptical of assumptions that taking part in interviews or group discussions can be therapeutic. While this may be true for some persons, it is better to admit that this is unpredictable and that some may be distressed by partaking. The information leaflet, like the study protocol, should give details about arrangements to help participants distressed in this way.

For most qualitative studies, participants should be offered ample time to consider whether to take part, and they should be offered the information leaflet to take away for further deliberation. For all but emergency research, committees generally insist that participants are given at least twenty-four hours to deliberate. They are usually not persuaded by requests to waive this on grounds of inconvenience or difficulty with recruitment. The leaflet should contain the name and contact details of the investigator, in case a potential participant needs further information or clarification when deliberating.

In addition to information sharing, the information leaflet should state clearly that taking part is voluntary. There should be an assurance that refusal to participate will not affect the standard of the person's clinical care. The leaflet should use neutral, descriptive language, and this may be a challenge to the investigator who naturally feels passionate about her study. The temptation to say that the study is vitally important, and that the supervisor is a world expert in the field, should be resisted. These may be true, but saying so can be coercive.

Whether subjects should be rewarded for taking part is controversial (Lavender and Briscoe, 2000), and different ethics committees take differing views on this. The majority view is that inducements should not be offered, and that participants should only be refunded travel and other expenses. In some studies modest rewards, such as gift vouchers to teenagers, may be appropriate if taking part involves substantial inconvenience or commitment, but they should be seen as recompense for this, not as an aid to recruitment, and rewards should not be so great as to persuade people to take part in research that might be against their best interests.

Confidentiality

The participant information leaflet, and the study protocol, should outline clearly how data will be obtained, including the use of audio or video recording. They should describe the measures planned to protect confidentiality, such as secure storage of notes and recordings, disposal of these after the study is completed and measures to protect the identity of participants when the findings are presented and published.

Investigators must appreciate that research ethics committees do not provide legal advice, and that ethical approval of their project does not absolve them from their legal responsibilities. Investigators are responsible for familiarising themselves with, and complying with, the requirements of the Data Protection Act (Department of Health, 2000), and Caldicott regulations governing access to patient records (Department of Health, 1998).

Interpreting and publishing the study findings

Disseminating the findings of good quality research is an ethical imperative. It can be disappointing to see that the summit of an investigator's ambition is to complete her Master's dissertation, and one often wonders whether, with a bit more effort in planning and writing up the study, a wider audience might not benefit from wider dissemination. To recruit subjects to a small project with the purposes of practising research and of getting a degree could be viewed from a Kantian perspective as using the subjects as means to these ends. Arguably, good quality research has the higher ends of educating society, and possibly benefiting present and future patients, and these ends might be approached by aiming higher than just writing the dissertation.

I have already discussed the ethical importance of integrity in writing up the research findings. This should be self-evident, but the temptations to report selectively, perhaps to reinforce prior assumptions or preconceptions, can be great. Publishing misleading research findings is unethical from both consequentialist and deontological standpoints.

Conclusions

In my view the stated ethical differences between quantitative and qualitative research are simply differences of degree and emphasis. Qualitative researchers in health care have ethical responsibilities to conduct methodologically sound research, to seek informed consent, to protect participants from harm associated with the research, to protect participant confidentiality and to disseminate the research findings honestly. These same principles also govern ethical quantitative research.

Suggestions for further reading

Many of the books cited in the reference list are a rich source of further reading in medical ethics (Beauchamp and Childress, Gillon, Hope *et al*), research ethics (Doyal and Tobias, Eckstein), and qualitative research (Denzin and Lincoln, Murphy *et al*).

Healthcare researchers should familiarise themselves with the Department of Health's 2001 research governance framework. The literature in these areas is vast. Here are a few suggestions for relevant further reading not already referred to.

Dickenson D (2002) *Ethical Issues in Maternal-Fetal Medicine.* Cambridge University Press, Cambridge

Giacomini M, Cook D (2000) 'Users' guides to the medical literature. XXIII. Qualitative research in health care. A. Are the results of the study valid?' *JAMA* **284**: 357–62.
One of a large series of articles in *JAMA* on critical appraisal of the medical literature.

Pope C, Campbell R (2001) 'Qualitative research in obstetrics and gynaecology'. *Br J Obstet Gynaecol* **108**: 233–37
A very useful overview, containing many illustrative examples of research projects.

Mauthner M, Birch M, Jessop J, Miller T (2002) *Ethics in Qualitative Research.* Sage, London
This book gives a detailed account of the practical ethical dilemmas experienced in the field by qualitative researchers. The feminist perspective is relevant to participants and researchers in qualitative research in midwifery and obstetrics.

References

Beauchamp T, Childress J (2001) *Principles of Biomedical Ethics.* 5th edn. Oxford University Press, Oxford

Beecher, H (1966) Ethics and clinical research. *N Engl J Medicine* **274**: 1354–60

Caplan A (1992) When evil intrudes. *Hastings Center Report* **22**(6): 29–32

Chalmers I, Lindley R. (2001) Double standards on informed consent to treatment. In: Doyal L, Tobias J, eds. *Informed Consent in Medical Research.* BMJ Books, London

Cribb A (2003) Approaching qualitative research. In: Eckstein S, ed. *Manual for Research Ethics Committees.* Cambridge University Press, Cambridge

Department of Health (1998) *Implementing the recommendations of the Caldicott report.* DoH, London

Department of Health (2000) *Data Protection Act 1998. Protection and Use of Patient Information.* DoH, London

Department of Health (2001a) *The research governance framework for health and social care.* DoH, London

Department of Health (2001b) *Governance arrangements for NHS research ethics committees.* DoH, London

Doyal L, Tobias J, eds (2001) *Informed Consent in Medical Research.* BMJ Books, London

Eckstein S, ed (2003) *Manual for Research for Ethics Committees.* CUP, Cambridge

Gillon R (1986) *Philosophical Medical Ethics.* John Wiley & Sons, Chichester

Green J (1999) Commentary: generalisability and validity in qualitative research. *Br Med J* **319**: 421

Hope T, Savulescu J, Kendrick J (2003) *Medical Ethics and Law. The core curriculum.* Churchill Livingstone, London

Lavender T, Briscoe L (2000) Research incentives: a thank you or a bribe? *Br J Midwif* **8**(4): 206

Mays N, Pope C (2000) Assessing quality in qualitative research. *Br Med J* **320**: 50–2

Mill JS (1991) *On Liberty and Other Essays*. Oxford University Press, Oxford

Murphy E, Dingwall R, Greatbatch D, Parker S, Watson P (1998) Qualitative research methods in health technology assessment: a review of the literature. *Health Technol Assess* **2**(16)

Papworth M (1967) *Human Guinea Pigs*. Routledge and Kegan Paul, London

Punch M (1998) Ethics and politics in qualitative research. In: Denzin N, Lincoln Y, eds. *The Landscape of Qualitative Research*. Sage, London

Ramcharan P, Cutcliffe J (2001) Judging the ethics of qualitative research: considering the 'ethics as process' model. *Health Soc Care in the Community* **9**(6) 358–66

Rosenhan D (1973) On being sane in insane places. *Science* **179**: 250–58

Rothman D (1987) Ethics and human experimentation. Henry Beecher revisited. *N Engl J Med* **317**: 1195–99

Shuster E (1997) Fifty years later: the significance of the Nuremberg Code. *N Engl J Med* **337**: 1436–40

World Medical Association Declaration of Helsinki (2000) *Ethical principles for Medical Research Involving Human Subjects*. WHO, Geneva

Chapter 4

Planning your research

Jane Morgan

The whole of science is nothing more than a refinement of everyday thinking.
Albert Einstein, 1879–1955

Considerations before you start? Introduction

Qualitative research is exciting and important as it enables us to understand what matters to women and why. Mason (2002: 1) advocates qualitative research as it enables researchers to explore the dimensions of the social world, which includes 'the texture and weave of everyday life, the understandings, experiences, and imaginings of our research participants' in the context of institutions, social processes, relationships and the significance and the meanings they generate. For the midwife or obstetrician wishing to undertake a piece of research, a qualitative approach provides an opportunity to gain insight not only into the experience of the participant, which may be staff or consumer, but also the context in which care is delivered in, which may be hospital or community. Whereas quantitative research sets out to test theory, qualitative research generates theory, and is useful when wanting to find out about thoughts, feelings or experiences of individuals, or when there is little known about a subject or concept. It is beneficial to midwives and obstetricians as it can provide valuable insight into what women actually experience during their contact with the maternity service. But perhaps more importantly, the findings of such research can be directly beneficial to women, who deserve to have the best evidence made available to them in order to make informed choices. This concept was endorsed in the Changing Childbirth Report (Department of health [DoH], 1993) in which choice, control, and continuity were advocated for women accessing maternity services. Kirkham (1994) likens the skills of qualitative research, listening and observation, to those skills required by the midwife. Although qualitative research has been a popular research methodology with some midwifery researchers for many years, it is now starting to find a place within the medical profession, as is witnessed by its infiltration into medical journals. Pope and Mays (1995) published a series of articles in the *British Medical Journal* that set out to describe qualitative research and its value in healthcare research. Likewise, Alderson (1998), in the same journal, discussed the importance of theories and values in health research. Tension often exists between the two approaches with conflict over the weighting and importance given to quantitative and qualitative research within clinical practice. Both approaches are appropriate within maternity care as both have strengths and weaknesses, and should be conducted in the same systematic, rigorous and transparent manner.

It is the intention of this chapter to take you through the process of how you can go about turning your good idea into a workable research question/statement using a qualitative approach. Factors you will need to consider at the outset of your research journey, such as resources, literature review, design, will be addressed.

Getting started

Finding a focus for the research is often difficult, despite the midwife or obstetrician having an idea of a subject area to research. The research question has to be developed from this broad focus, enabling the researcher to progress through the study in a planned and rigorous way. The development of the research question is crucial; as it is on this that all stages of the research process depend. The midwife or obstetrician may generate ideas for research by reflection and analysis on their clinical practice or by reading and reviewing literature. The clinician's own working environment often instigates the research focus. It may be that a new development has been introduced into clinical practice, or there may be some concern regarding current practice. Research in clinical practice should aim to improve maternity services and care to women and their families so it is important when finding an area of focus for research that the issue of relevance is considered. Rees (1997) states that the contribution the research makes to midwifery could be in terms of increasing knowledge in practice, generating or testing theory or informing policy. Before embarking on their own piece of research, midwives and obstetricians should ask themselves of what benefit there would be to women and/ or their babies and families? Once a decision has been made that the research should be carried out, the next stage is to work out how it should be done.

Understanding the influences on how the research is carried out

Apart from being clear about the theoretical perspective (discussed in *Chapter 2*), other factors impinge on the qualitative research process, such as values and practical issues (Bryman, 2001).

Research values

Values reflect the personal beliefs and feelings of the researcher and there is growing recognition that it is not feasible to expect the researcher to hold these feelings in check. Suspending one's feelings in research is known as 'bracketing'. It is therefore inevitable that they will impinge on the research. This can occur at numerous opportunities during the research process. Researcher bias may occur in a qualitative study at any time point, from choice of research question to interpretation of analysis. Furthermore, it has been known for researchers to develop an affinity or sympathy towards their participants if engaged in intense data collection technique with them. A researcher exploring the views of women suffering from domestic violence, for example, may become so immersed in the data that they have difficulty suspending their own beliefs. A good qualitative researcher will acknowledge that the research cannot be value free, demonstrate reflexivity and take adequate steps to minimise bias.

Qualitative research usually requires a high level of engagement and interaction from the researcher. In order to do this the researcher needs to develop skills to enable him/her to identify the key issues of the research, working out how to solve them and being able to understand the intellectual, practical, moral and political implications of resolving them (Mason, 2002). Throughout the research process the researcher should employ a self-questioning approach, and it is these reflexive acts that become an integral part of the whole research process. What this means is that because the researcher is not neutral or detached from the knowledge and evidence gathering, the researcher needs to reflect on his or her role in the research process and the impact this may have. It is acceptable practice for the researcher to demonstrate how any of their own biases and assumptions has informed the research and its subsequent findings. Thomson (1995), in her study of maternal behaviour during spontaneous and directed pushing in the second stage of labour, reported that two midwives commented that had the researcher not been there observing the birth, both midwives would have been tempted to tell the woman to take a deep breath and resort to directed pushing despite the woman being allocated to the spontaneous pushing group. The researcher's presence in the field, or labour ward in this case, clearly has an influence on the research and the 'social actors', ie. the midwives. It is this type of tension that needs to be addressed throughout the qualitative research process.

Practical issues of research

Practical issues include decisions on how the research should be carried out and the resources available to the researcher (*Figure 4.1*).

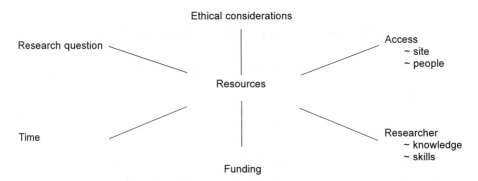

Figure 4.1: Practical considerations

It is important to pay attention to these issues when planning your research proposal as addressing them at the start of the research will ultimately save you time and help for a smooth running research project.

The researcher

Midwives and obstetricians may vary from the novice to the expert researcher. However, regardless of research competence, he or she must demonstrate his/her competence to conduct a thorough, ethical piece of qualitative research (*Chapter 3*). It would be considered unacceptable for a researcher to embark on conducting a randomised controlled trial without taking advice from experienced trialists; similarly, it is unacceptable to conduct a piece of qualitative research without seeking relevant expertise. Midwives and obstetricians sometimes confuse their clinical observational and interviewing skills with the ability to perform qualitative research, yet these skills are not the same. The qualitative researcher must have a good understanding of the theory, methodology and methods of the approach and should demonstrate this with clear and explicit protocols.

The growing interest in qualitative research has led to an abundance of avenues from which novice researchers can obtain help, advice and supervision. The research may be a requirement of an academic programme such as MPhil or PhD, in which case a supervisory team will be appointed and the researcher, as part of the course requirement, would undertake methodology training. If the researcher does not have academic supervision, help should be sought from the Trust research and development department. Professional bodies or voluntary organisations may be interested and increasingly, collaborative studies are being encouraged between clinicians and academia as a way of achieving effective clinical research.

Funding

Funding can be difficult to obtain and in comparison with other types of health-related research, there is no doubt that qualitative research is not as widely funded, but it is a myth that government agencies and medical charities do not fund qualitative research. As with any other type of research funding, applications may be unsuccessful due to an applicant's insufficient knowledge of field, choice of an inappropriate methodology to answer their research question, a poorly written application form, or unrealistic cost and time projections. Qualitative research is frequently more time-consuming than quantitative research, and this should always be reflected in realistic cost projections to potential funders. Guidance for researchers planning to submit a funding application for qualitative research has improved in recent years, although it remains highly competitive. In 1999 the National Institutes for Health (NIH) in North America held a workshop entitled 'Qualitative Methods in Health Research: Opportunities and Considerations in Applications and Review', following which the Office of Behavioural and Social Sciences Research published guidance to assist researchers using qualitative methods in submitting competitive funding applications for support from NIH (http://www.nih.gov/icd/). There are regional and national research and development bodies such as the Medical Research Council (MRC) and it is worth visiting the RD Info Health Related website which offers a range of funding bodies (www.rdinfo.org.uk).

Time

The length of time it takes from having the 'good idea' to formulating the research proposal and carrying out the research through to the dissemination phase usually takes far longer than anticipated. There may be an enforced time frame if you are undertaking the research for further study, contracted by a funding body or working as part of an NHS Trust project, but whatever the reason for carrying out the research, it is important to have a formal and realistic time frame. Obtaining ethical approval can take months (see *Chapter 3*, for discussion on ethical approval), as can writing up the research so make sure that you build in enough time for each stage. Drawing up a timetable from when the research is to start and when it will end will ensure that all stages of the research process are covered. Many researchers use Gant charts such as the one illustrated in *Figure 4.2.*

	1	2	3	4	5	6	7	8	9	10	11	12	13	14	15	16	17	18
Ethical approval	X	X	X															
Recruitment				X	X	X	X											
Data collection					X	X	X	X	X									
Data analysis						X	X	X	X	X	X	X						
Report writing													X	X	X			
Dissemination																X	X	X

Figure 4.2: Example of an eighteen-month Gant chart

Access to participants/site

A further consideration is how to access potential research participants. Sampling is discussed further on in the chapter but it is still important at this early stage to consider the practical issues of site access and participants. If the researcher is not employed in the research site then it is necessary to gain managerial approval to conduct the research in that trust. This is often done through the research and development department. In some units, the researcher will require an honorary contract to enable them to work as a researcher in that trust; this means that health clearance has to be gained from occupational health. A search may also be required from the Criminal Records Bureau (police search), all of which adds time and possible delay to starting your research. I was recently called to the occupational health department of a trust for a medical just to obtain an honorary trust contract as a researcher. The occupational nurse, on discovering that I would not be having patient contact while undertaking my research project, nor did I require a medical examination, decided to test my eyes so I didn't have a wasted visit! All of this delayed my obtaining the necessary contract to set foot in the trust in order to collect my data.

Research question/statement

The research question or statement chosen will influence which research strategy will be utilised. In order to find out about sensitive issues or illicit activities such as drug taking in pregnancy, it would be more practical and appropriate to use a qualitative approach, which would enable the researcher to develop a relationship and rapport with the participants in order to gain insight and understanding into their experiences. Unlike quantitative research, which proposes a hypothesis, which is then tested by accepting or rejecting this proposed theory, qualitative research does not have a proposed theory but aims to generate theory from the data. This 'inductive' process is aiming to describe and give meaning to how the participants in the research give meaning to their world. This means that the research question in qualitative research may be in the form of a question or a statement or an aim. For example, your clinical interest may be 'normal childbirth' and you may want to find out about women's experiences of normal childbirth. This would lend itself to a qualitative research strategy that would enable the researcher to elicit the views of this particular group of women in an exploratory way. The overall aim or statement of intent of the research could be about women's experiences of birth and from this you may want to have some specific questions or statements you wish your research to address. However, often the research question/statement will change, or become more refined following a review of the literature so it is best to leave the specificity of the research statement until after you have completed such a review. This also applies to how you will design your research, meaning which methodology will you select that will enable you to best answer the research question.

Literature review

Having now identified a subject area to focus on it is important to carry out a review of the literature. The purpose of this is:

1. To find out what is already known about the subject area and are there any gaps in the knowledge?
2. How is it known? How have other researchers gone about their research? What methodology and methods have been used?
3. To assist in formulating your research question and choosing an appropriate research strategy.
4. To develop a conceptual framework for the research.

Accessing the literature is time-consuming and can often be frustrating, but a thorough search of the literature should be carried out to provide a comprehensive overview of the subject. The search process should involve accessing primary and secondary sources of literature. Primary sources include journals, published original studies, clinical guidelines, systematic reviews, case reports, published reports, trials and research registers, bulletins, newsletters and conference proceedings. Primary sources also include 'grey' literature, which include theses, dissertations, and newsletters. Secondary sources include commentaries and editorials on the subject or on the primary sources. The methodology of literature search has changed considerably since the growth of the Internet that has transformed the way literature can be accessed and disseminated. Although literature sources can be accessed directly via a library, database searching is an essential component of the literature search. For midwifery there are specific bibliographic services such as MIRIAD, Midwives and Information and Research Service (MIDIRS), Royal College of Midwives (RCM) Current Awareness Service, Cochrane Pregnancy and Childbirth Database. For obstetricians and for health in general, there are databases such as PUBMED, MEDLINE, CINAHL, BNI, PsychLIT. Snowball (1999: 34–46) provides a select list of information resources.

To conduct a thorough literature search it is necessary to be organised and systematic in your approach. Provided that you search through all the key strategies, eg. electronic databases, library catalogues, book bibliographies, current awareness services, abstracting and indexing journals, special indexes, it does not matter in which order you do it. Once you have started the process of retrieving the literature you have the task of reading it, identifying themes within the subject area and recording what you have read. For example, a literature search on normal birth will identify a vast amount of literature which can be themed into categories such as 'place of birth', 'midwifery practice', 'obstetrician's practice', 'maternal morbidity', 'fetal outcomes', 'monitoring in labour', and so on. It is good practice to develop a system of recording what you are reading, the full reference, and details of the content. There are various ways of organising this system, such as using index cards in author, subject, alphabetical or date order (see Burton, 2000:137–152 for examples of manual paper-based system) or a software package such as Reference Manager or Endnote. It is well worth developing this skill, as not only does it help you to organise your thoughts and reading, it saves time when it comes to finding references that you need for your bibliography. Reading the literature can sometimes be tedious, as it is not the same as reading a novel where the reader is enticed into a story by having their thoughts and senses stimulated. Developing the art of skim reading is essential in order to decide whether the particular article is worth reading in more depth using critical reading skills. Critical reading involves reflecting on the significance of the work, asking questions about its strengths and weaknesses, how does it relate to other pieces of work? Does it inform, or have the potential to inform clinical practice? Not only do you apply this approach to what the piece of work is saying or concluding, but also how it is able to say it, ie. what methodology or approach has been used? Are there any flaws in the process? Was it an appropriate approach? What theoretical ideas have underpinned the piece of work? By doing this you will be able to structure the review into a framework to present the existing knowledge that may then enable you to identify where there is a gap in the knowledge, or if there is a 'gap' in the way the knowledge has been obtained. This means that there could be another way of researching this subject, which hasn't yet been carried out, which may give a different perspective or a deeper understanding of the subject area.

Research question/statement

From this immersion in the literature, there is now the process of refining the focus and formulating the research question/statement. Mason (2002: 14) suggests five important questions that will help the researcher to articulate what the very essence of their research is about:

1. What is the nature of the phenomena, or entities, or social reality that I wish to investigate? (the social reality: your ontological perspective?)
2. What might represent knowledge or evidence of the entities or 'social reality' that I wish to investigate? (knowledge and evidence: your epistemological position?)

3. What topic, or broad substantive area, is the research concerned with? (Your broad research area)
4. What is the intellectual puzzle? What do I wish to explain or explore? What type of puzzle is it?
5. What are my research questions?

These questions offer the researcher a framework to enable them to organise their thoughts and literature to formulate the research question(s).

Silverman (2000) highlights the difficulty in narrowing down your research area when drafting a research proposal and cites Wolcott (1990: 62), 'do less, more thoroughly'. This is good advice as often the researcher is so immersed in the literature that it is difficult to see out of the 'fog' this immersion generates. Silverman (2000: 67) offers three practical techniques:

- draw a flow chart
- find a puzzle
- look through a zoom lens.

Flow chart

Drawing a flow chart to help relate the key concepts to the study will help to formulate key research questions to deal with the data generated in the analysis stage. A single page flow chart (*Figure 4.3*), or plan (*Figure 4.4*), provides a point of reference separate to your working document and is a useful technique in moving from a broad research focus to a clearly defined research question. Without this clearly defined research question, data analysis will be very difficult and unwieldy.

Finding the puzzle

Another way of moving out of the 'fog' of the literature is to set the books and reading to one side and ask yourself, 'What is it I am trying to find out? What puzzle am I trying to solve?' Silverman (2000) cites Mason (1996) who describes this as the intellectual puzzle around which all qualitative research should be formulated and denotes three categories of the puzzle:

'How or why did X develop? (developmental puzzle)
How does X work? (mechanical puzzle)
What causes X or what influence does X have on Y? (causal puzzle)'

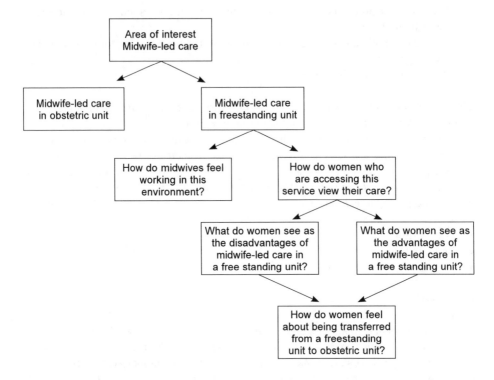

Figure 4.3: Flow chart to illustrate the refining of research questions

To relate this framework to a research area, the midwife may have an interest in women who use illegal substances in pregnancy. The questions in the puzzle could be:

- How was illegal substance use in pregnancy first recognised? (a developmental puzzle)
- How are the women who use illegal substances in pregnancy identified, and by whom? (mechanical puzzle)
- What are the characteristics of the women who use illegal substances in pregnancy?
- What effect do the illegal substances have on women, on their pregnancy and on the baby? (causal puzzle).

This focusing down onto specific puzzles then enables the midwife to be even more specific and able to choose one of the puzzles depending on a number of factors; such as which puzzle is the more interesting to the midwife, which does she have the most literature, knowledge or experience of, which aspect of the puzzle is the funding body most interested in? These considerations demonstrate how the formulation of the research question is a process subjected to many influences.

Aim: To explore women's views of home birth

Statement of intent: An exploratory study to explore the views of women on home birth

Research question: What are women's views of homebirth?

[After a literature search, one may discover that the home birth rate is particularly low amongst a particular population]

Refined question: Why is the home birth rate amongst Asian women in Blackburn so low?

[To add multiple perspectives the question is further refined into more specific questions, which will require a triangulated, approach (see *Chapter 5*)]

Primary question: What are the internal and external factors, which are influencing the low home birth rate amongst Asian women in Blackburn?

Secondary questions:

❖ What are the views of Asian women on home birth?

❖ What cultural factors may be influencing Asian womens' decisions to give birth at home?

❖ What are the views of midwives who are working with Asian women?

[These secondary questions will assist with deciding on appropriate methods. For example, to answer question 1, interviews or focus groups may be conducted. To answer question 2, interviews may be conducted with family members and/or observations within the home environment may be conducted. Similarly, to answer question 3, the researcher may observe the midwife/woman interaction at home or hospital or she may question a sample of midwives using one-to-one interviews or focus groups. The actual approach will be determined by the researchers theoretical perspective as discussed in *Chapter 2*.]

Figure 4.4: A plan to refine research questions

Zoom lens

The zoom lens analogy is about enabling the researcher to first of all look at the big picture, then zoom in onto one particular aspect or unit of the picture. The bigger the picture, the less fine the detail. For the midwife or obstetrician who is interested in women who use illegal substances in pregnancy, the zoom in could be one woman, or one antenatal clinic for the women, or one birth experience. Using this approach the midwife can always revert back to the bigger picture to keep a perspective on the research.

The research statement/aim/questions should be original and grounded in an understanding of the literature. They should express the 'essence' of the research. They should also be open enough to allow you to explore further and ask further questions as you generate data and analysis. The question(s) should be clearly formulated, as it is through the questions that you will be 'joining what you are going to research' with 'how you are going to do it'.

Designing your qualitative study

There is often confusion between the terms 'methodology' and 'methods'. Cluett and Bluff (2000: 213) define methodology as 'the theoretical beliefs, or the perspective on which the study is based'. This means the theory behind how the research should be carried out. Silverman (2000) states that methodology is a general approach to studying research topics, ie. it is how the researcher goes about studying the topic. Methods are specific research techniques, or tools, that are used within the study to collect the data. It could be a questionnaire that the respondent completes or it could be an unstructured interview. There are many different methods used to collect the data. The research design is the framework or plan of how the study is to be carried out. The main steps in carrying out qualitative research are less defined than in quantitative research. Bryman (2001: 264) highlights the five main preoccupation of qualitative research:

1. Seeing through the eyes of the participants
2. Description and context
3. Process
4. Flexibility and lack of structure
5. Concepts and theory as outcomes of the research process.

These five main areas need to be considered when thinking about how best to address your research questions and what approach to take to do so.

What you want the research question/statement to explore or discover will determine which qualitative methodology will be the most appropriate to do this. Other chapters in this book (see *Chapter 2*) elaborate on the different qualitative approaches and for additional reading see Creswell (1998), in his book *Qualitative Inquiry and Research Design*. Choosing among five traditions provides critical analysis and discussion on five qualitative traditions of inquiry: biography, phenomenology, grounded theory, ethnography, and case study.

Sampling

As the research outcome is dependent on a carefully designed research approach, the selection of the sample is crucial, as an inappropriate sample can adversely affect the outcome of the research. It is important to consider carefully whom you will need to study in order to answer your research question.

In order to discuss the types of sampling relevant to qualitative research we need to clarify what 'population' and 'sample' mean. Rees (1997: 133) defines population as, 'the total group of people, things or events the researcher is interested in saying something about.' In other words, it is a specified group that shares a common set of characteristics. The sample, therefore, is a component of this group or population.

In quantitative research the size of the sample is often large in order to test hypotheses and provide valid and reliable results that are generalisable. The sample frame is established before the research begins. However, in qualitative research, which is seeking to find out about the experiences of individuals in relation to particular phenomena, the sample size is small and will generate a considerable amount of in-depth data. Those recruited to a qualitative study are selected as they represent a particular group and recruitment follows a different set of rules compared with quantitative research design.

The most commonly cited types of sample associated with qualitative research are purposive, convenience, snowball, and theoretical (Rees, 1997; Cluett and Bluff, 2000; Bryman, 2001). For information on other sampling strategies such as random, purposeful, opportunistic or critical case, refer to Marshall and Rossman (1999).

Purposive sampling

This allows the researcher to select the people who have the experience or knowledge of the topic the researcher is studying. Purposive sampling is about seeking out groups or individuals where the processes studied are likely to occur. Silverman (2000) highlights the need to think carefully and critically about who is selected and how this selection takes place, especially within the constraints of research resources. You may wish to study the experiences of midwives who have assisted women in home birth. It would not be possible to research every midwife so you need to decide whether to select a group of midwives from the same geographical area or a smaller group from two different geographical areas. It is important to justify the selection process and ensure that this is evident to ensure transparency in the research. Rees (1997) suggests that while there is potential researcher bias to this approach, the very opposite will be achieved if the researcher strives to include participants with a range of the experience. Purposive sampling is well suited to a phenomenological approach as it enables the researcher to recruit those who have experienced the phenomena in question. For example, in Briscoe and Streets' (2003) work which explored 'vanishing twins', the findings would have lacked meaning if the women interviewed had not actually experienced a 'vanished twin'.

Convenience sampling

Convenience sampling refers to individuals who are easily accessible to the researcher and is useful as long as those individuals have the necessary experience or knowledge of the subject. For example, a researcher may recruit women attending antenatal clinic on a particular day or obstetricians attending a professional conference. A limitation of this strategy occurs when the researcher is only available at certain times to recruit individuals into the study resulting in a biased sample. Cluett (2000) notes that research has to be carried out in the real world so sometimes this problem is unavoidable. It is, however, important to acknowledge this. Convenience sampling can be used in phenomenological research and ethnography where the researcher is setting out to study those in that particular field or setting.

Snowball sampling

In snowball sampling, also referred to as chain or nominated sampling, individuals relevant to the study provide details of others that may be useful to include in the study. It is useful in situations where the researcher is finding it difficult to identify individuals to take part in the study, or where there are difficulties in gaining access to the individuals where anonymity may be desirable. For example, the researcher may be having difficulty in finding women who have experienced postnatal depression. One woman in this situation may know of others perhaps from attending a support group. Salmon (1999) uses this technique to recruit women into a qualitative study to explore their experiences of childbirth and perineal trauma. Each participant referred someone to the researcher until the sample size was achieved. While this is a useful way to recruit women, its weakness lies in the fact that the sample may be from a similar background with similar characteristics and outlook.

Theoretical sampling

Cluett and Bluff (2000: 216) define theoretical sampling as 'sampling that is determined by concepts, categories and emerging theory that is grounded in the data'.

This means that theoretical sampling is a way of selecting the sample and a way of knowing when to stop gathering data. Within the grounded theory approach Strauss and Corbin (1998) suggest open sampling to begin with. The researcher collects and analyses data from sources, which are of interest to the study, such as interviewing participants, observing events or studying documents. Theoretical sampling takes place from this data collection and analysis to identify the emerging issues. This process enables the researcher to identify new participants in the development of theory. The data collection continues until no more new theories emerge. This point in the study is known as theoretical or data saturation. In theoretical sampling it is not possible to predict at the beginning of the study what size the sample will be as the size may change during the course of the research study. Mason (1996) describes this flexibility as being able to manipulate analysis, theory and sampling in an interactive way. This flexibility will allow you to seek out other individuals for your study as new factors emerge.

Sample size is generally small in qualitative research and Holloway and Wheeler (1996) suggest a range from four to fifty participants, although they do acknowledge that it is not the size of the study that is of relevance but the process.

With regard to selecting your sample you need to consider:

- your chosen approach to the research
- who are the appropriate individuals?
- how will you access them?
- what kind of sampling strategy will you use?
- can you justify this?
- are there any ethical considerations in recruiting this sample?

Trustworthiness

Trustworthiness is about ensuring that qualitative research represents the truth. Qualitative research is concerned primarily with seeing through the eyes of the participants. An important feature of qualitative research is to provide description of the setting the research takes place in, with emphasis on the context in order to understand the social world of the participants. There is also emphasis on process which provides insight into how events and/or patterns occur during the course of the research. In order to achieve this it is necessary to have a fairly unstructured approach to the data collection. This enables the researcher some flexibility should there be a need to change direction during the research study. This contrasting approach to how quantitative research is carried out has been criticised by quantitative researchers. Their main argument is that such an approach is too subjective, being dependent on the views of the researcher as to what is important. Further criticism is that it is difficult to replicate the study, and not possible to generalise the findings to other settings outside of the small group in which the research was conducted.

Conclusion

In summary, Marshall and Rossman (1999) suggest that the research proposal in a qualitative research study comprise of three components:

1. The introduction, which gives an overview of the proposal, the topic area, the research questions, the study's purpose and significance and any limitations.
2. The literature, a discussion of the literature which informs the study and its place in the current discourse around the subject area, including its theoretical traditions.
3. Research design and methods, detailing sample population or site of interest, methods for gathering data and analysing the data, how 'trustworthiness' will be ensured, and any other political or ethical issues which may impinge on the study.

This chapter addresses how your initial idea, which may have arisen from a hunch in clinical practice, an experience, observation or a personal theory, has motivated you to investigate it further leading you to decide whether it would be just and right to conduct research in that area. From deciding that it 'should be done' the chapter takes you through some of the issues and practicalities of 'getting it started', making decisions about how you want to start to build your research framework with subsequent chapters exploring the further stages in the qualitative research process.

References

Alderson P (1998) The importance of theories in healthcare. *Br Med J* **317**: 1007–10

Briscoe L, Street C (2003) 'Vanished Twin': An exploration of women's experiences. *Birth* **30**: 47–53

Bryman A (2001) *Social Research Methods*. Oxford University Press, Oxford

Burton D (2000) Using literature to support research. In Burton D, ed. *Research Training for Social Scientists*. Sage, London: 37–152

Cluett ER (2000) Experimental Research. In Cluett ER, Bluff R, eds. *Principles and Practice of Research in Midwifery*. Baillière Tindall, London

Cluett ER, Bluff R, eds (2000) *Principles and Practice of Research in Midwifery*. Baillière Tindall, London

Creswell JW (1998) *Qualitative Inquiry and Research Design. Choosing among five traditions*. Sage, London: 47–72

Department of Health (1993) *Report of the Expert Maternity Committee Group: Changing Childbirth*. HMSO, London

Holloway I, Wheeler S (1996) *Qualitative Research for Nursing*. Blackwell Science, Oxford

Kirkham M (1994) Using research skills in midwifery practice. *Br J Midwif* 2(8): 390–92

Marshall C, Rossman GB (1999) *Designing Qualitative Research*. 3rd edn. Sage, London

Mason J (2002) *Qualitative Researching*. 2nd edn. Sage, London

Mason J (1996) Qualitative researching. In Silverman D, ed. *Doing Qualitative Research. A Practical Handbook*. Sage, London

Pope C, Mays N (1995) Reaching the parts other methods cannot reach: an introduction to qualitative methods in health and health services research. *Br Med J* **311**: 42–5

Rees C (1997) *An Introduction to Research for Midwives*. Books for Midwives, Oxford

Salmon D (1999) A feminist analysis of women's experiences of perineal trauma in the immediate post-delivery period. *Midwifery* **15**: 247–56

Silverman D (2000) *Doing Qualitative Research. A Practical Handbook*. Sage, London

Snowball R (1999) Finding the evidence: an information skills approach. In: Dawes M, Davies P, Gray A, Mant J, Seers K, Snowball R, eds. *Evidence-based Practice. A Primer for Health Care Professionals*. Churchill Livingstone, Edinburgh

Strauss A, Corbin J (1998) *Basics of Qualitative Research Techniques and Procedures for Developing Grounded Theory*. 2nd edn, Sage, California

Thomson AM (1995) Maternal behaviour during spontaneous and directed pushing in the second stage of labour. *J Adv Nurs* **22**: 1027–34

Wolcott HF (1990) *Writing up Qualitative Research*. Sage Publications, Newbury Park

Chapter 5

How to collect qualitative data

Denis Walsh and Lisa Baker

The more interactions we ascertain, the more we know the object in question.
John Dewey, 1859–1952

Introduction

Data collection in qualitative research is evolving all the time. Though interviews and observation have been and remain the principal methods of data collection, over the last ten years a variety of other approaches have begun to be utilised including text mediums like narrative, written records, internet, email and visual mediums like film, video, photo and drawing.

This chapter will concentrate mainly on interviews, both one-to-one and focus groups, observation and diaries, as these remain the most widely used within health care. However, alternative and novel approaches like text and visual mediums will also be introduced. The advent of these approaches is linked to the realisation that knowledge generation associated with qualitative research, can be communicated in a variety of ways. This is because qualitative research understands knowledge as constructed, not objectively 'true' and contingent on the context of investigation.

Anthropology is credited with the origins of interviews and participant observation. Both techniques were used as the classic way of studying alternative, usually indigenous, cultures. Famous anthropologists like Mead and Malinowski championed them over eighty years ago as the primary data collection methods of ethnography (Holloway and Wheeler, 1996). Ethnography is the study of cultures and is a key method approach within the paradigm of qualitative research. Sociologists adapted the in-depth interview and participant observation in the 1960s to explore subcultures like gangs and homelessness within Western societies and, since that time, health professionals have extended its application. Particularised ethnographies (Leininger, 1985) or the study of micro cultures like consultant delivery suites (Hunt and Symonds, 1995) or out patient clinics (Danziger, 1979) have grown exponentially over the past twenty years.

Interviews

The role of the research interview in maternity care is powerfully illustrated by Salmon (1999). She wanted to discover what were the important issues for women around care of the perineum during childbirth. Obstetricians and midwives have actually done quite a bit of research in this area with two Cochrane reviews on suture material and suture method (Kettle, 2003a; Kettle, 2003b) and the high profile multi-centre HOOP trial (McCandlish *et al*, 1998). All these studies share one crucial omission in their methods — an evaluation of a maternal perspective on the various interventions tested. Salmon's interviews revealed a completely different set of interests to what the professionals had investigated. Women's concerns were far more practical:

⌘ How can I have confidence that the person stitching my perineum is competent?
⌘ A positive rapport with this person is crucial to ensuring that the procedure is done with dignity and sensitivity.

Many of them spoke out of a bitter experience where there was incompetence and insensitivity.

Salmon's findings bring home to us the importance of not just involving women users in the evaluation of specific childbirth interventions but of also consulting with them when drawing up the research agenda. The interview is an effective way of addressing both these priorities.

Interviews provide more than just data on the experience of a childbirth intervention. They can also reveal the process of constructing meaning as childbirth events unfold. An appreciation of assigning meaning to life events is important for a number of reasons. Within a practice milieu that aims for clinical care to be evidence-based, 'meaning making' equates to Sackett *et al*'s (1996) 'patient compliance/preference' in his evidence triad. Sackett *et al* always understood evidence-based care to be an amalgam of good quality research, clinical expertise and patient preference.

Second, 'meaning making' recognises that people do not passively respond to clinical interventions in a uniform, predictable and mechanistic way. All of us integrate physiological, psychological and, many would say, spiritual dimensions (Henery, 2003; Isaia *et al*, 1999) of our being as we actively create our responses to healthcare interventions. An exploration of meaning gives us a window into understanding these processes. However, the most compelling reason for health practitioners to tease out meanings is humanistic — to express compassion for those we care for. Listening to them and seeking to understand their personal life story so that we better match our interventions to their individual circumstances is fundamental to the professional care ethic.

Purpose of research interviews

Maykut and Morehouse (1994) define the purpose of the research interview as a 'conversation with a purpose'. They state that, '… most critical to being a skilled qualitative interviewer is deep and genuine curiosity about understanding another's experience' and involves 'moving beyond surface talk to a rich discussion of thoughts and feelings' (p. 81). The main purpose of the qualitative interview is to:

• explore the meanings/perceptions and interpretations that individuals assign to their experiences.

Additional purposes are to:

• research sensitive topics, eg. childbirth experience, that are less suited to the more impersonal and prescriptive questionnaires
• generate theory around complex areas of care, eg. maternity care where there maybe considerable variation in the packages of care

- test existing theory
- clarify terms and issues as a precursor to a quantitative study.

Marchant and Kenny, 2000

Types of interview

There are three types of interview: unstructured (sometimes called in-depth); semi-structured; and structured (Van Teijlingen and Ireland, 2003).

Semi-structured and unstructured interviews are the most common in qualitative research. The structured interview is usually conducted with a questionnaire that is investigating pre-set areas and topics. It has similarities to the quantitative survey and is predominantly utilised in this way. These require the development of an interview schedule that should be piloted first. The classic market survey commonly involves this approach. Structured interviews do not exclude the possibility of the use of unstructured questions but these are the prerogative of the interviewer, not the interviewee. Semi-structured interviews are conducted on the basis of a loose structure consisting of open-ended questions that define the area to be explored, at least initially, and from which the interviewer or interviewee may diverge in order to pursue an idea in more detail. In-depth interviews are less structured than this, and may cover only one or two issues. Both methods have a purpose that is not just to free research participants to talk about the topic unfettered from prescribed questions set by the interviewer, but actually gives the interviewee's control of where they want to take the topic. In this sense, the original research question has to be broad enough to encompass and enable the investigator to follow unexpected and unanticipated directions from the data. When I (DW) explored women's experience of caseload midwifery practice, the expected focus on the value of a known midwife during labour was subordinate to women's primary concern for their relationship with their midwives throughout all phases of their care. Their concerns effectively changed the focus of the study (Walsh, 1999).

Despite the open-endedness of semi-structured and unstructured interviews, the researcher continues to influence the focus, according to the emerging themes from the data, as interviews continue. This means that though a common introductory question will start every interview, subsequent prompt questions may differ from one interview to the next. There is a dynamic in operation here between researcher and research participant, in which they both shape the focus of enquiry. The unstructured interview does not mean that the researcher asks the first question and passively listens to the remainder of the interview with no more contribution than some encouraging nods. Almost always, further questions are required to draw the interviewee out, but these questions are spontaneous and are formulated in response to what is being communicated. This requires active listening and constant reflection — skills that will be elaborated on in the next section.

How to interview

Fundamental to the skills of the interviewer is a non-judgemental approach, respectful of differences in cultural and social conventions and values. Nothing is more undermining of disclosure in interview than the suspicion that the questioner is disapproving of what is being said. This is communicated as powerfully through non-verbal responses as through verbal ones, and requires a high level of insight from the interviewer so the effects of these differences are masked as far as possible (Hammersley and Atkinson, 1995). During research into schoolgirl friendships, Hey (2002) found out that she was thought to be variously a social worker, head teacher, social worker, police officer, probation officer and someone's mum. Only in her latter interviews did trust and openness become apparent and she became accepted as a researcher with a genuine interest in the girls' lives. A willingness to listen actively is also fundamental. Here the skills are similar to the counsellor who seeks to put their client at ease and to encourage the development of trust. An open posture, leaning forward and maintaining eye contact are integral to the active listening disposition.

Choice of venue for the interview is also important in putting the research participant at ease – ideally their home if acceptable to them or a neutral setting away from the researcher's place of work. The researcher's profession can also be relevant, especially if the interviewee aligns them with the establishment and is therefore less likely to be critical. Class, race and gender of the interviewer may all have effects on interviewee's responses and the researcher needs to consider carefully how these effects can be ameliorated or utilised to advantage. Even the choice of clothes can impact on the rapport building if it contributes to the discomfort of the interviewee. Hunt relates such an incident when she was interviewing midwives on a labour ward who assumed she was a doctor because she wore theatre clothes (Hunt and Symonds, 1995). Thoughtful attention to these details can smooth the way for a successful interview (Van Teijlingen and Ireland, 2003).

Prior to undertaking an interview, the selection of equipment is critical. Recording equipment must be able to be heard easily on playback. This cannot be emphasised enough as the work of transcribing is time-consuming and made frustratingly longer and less successful if conversations cannot be clearly heard. Always check the recording ability in advance so equipment is known to work well. Before leaving to undertake interviews make sure that there are enough tapes packed and batteries if mains power is not available. Finally, ensure distractions are minimised as far as possible — televisions, radios, stereos off, pets likely to create noise removed, etc and try interviewing at a time that the interviewee is least likely to be distracted by other demands, eg. phones, other people.

Anonymity and guarantees of confidentiality need clarifying before the interview starts. Initial conversations should be friendly and informal, aiming at establishing rapport and creating a relaxed ambience for the interview. Commence the interview with an open, rather than closed, question, eg. 'Could you tell me about...'. Carry a discrete interview schedule as a reminder of areas to be covered if required. The use of probes is essential for in-depth interviews to elicit detail and depth from the interviewee. Maykut and Morehouse (1994) classify these as:

- detail-orientated probes — who, what, where, when and how questions
- elaboration probes — nodding, silence, softly voicing 'un-huh' or 'tell me more about', 'can you give an example'
- clarification probes — to increase understanding, eg. 'I am not sure I understand what you mean', repeating back the interviewer's perception to check for accuracy.

The researcher should be open to intuitive impulses in pursuing certain lines of enquiry and remain open to unanticipated twists and turns in the content of the interview. In particular, the interviewer should be alert to the expression of feelings and emotions, as these are known to influence powerfully the construction of meaning and the interpretation of experience (Taylor, 2001). Though their expression may require sensitive handling, they often lead to insight for both parties.

Transition comments are statements that change the topic like, 'I'd like to leave that now and move on...'. Ending an interview with a 'catch-all question', eg. 'Is there anything else you would like to say about...', is helpful in drawing out other issues of importance to the research participant.

Finally, most authorities advise that interviews should not last much longer then one hour and that if more data is likely to be required from the interviewee, a repeat interview should be scheduled (Hammersley and Atkinson, 1995).

There are a number of common pitfalls in interviewing which are outlined by Field and Morse (1989). These include stage fright for interviewer or interviewee, counselling or teaching mode adopted by interviewer, receiving secret information (for example, suicide threats), presenting one's own perspective thus potentially biasing the interview and the inability of the interviewees to articulate their ideas, experiences or perceptions. I found this especially when interviewing women about their experiences of birth in midwifery-led units. The interviews of better-educated women and those with more than one child went on for longer and required far less prompting from me to elicit information. The following excerpt from a transcript is typical.

Interviewer:	*Could you tell about the baby's birth?*
Interviewee:	*It was great.*
Interviewer:	*What exactly was so great about it?*
Interviewee:	*I don't know, it was just really good.*
Interviewer:	*In what way?*
Interviewee:	*You know, it just happened...*

This kind of interaction requires the interviewer to be patient and to possess an ability to be comfortable with silence. Even then, the quality of data may be superficial compared with an articulate woman who has the ability to be reflective.

Addressing rigour

There are a number of important steps that help ensure rigour in analysis. Keeping an 'audit trail' is one (Holloway and Wheeler, 1996). This is an accurate record of the various stages of data collection and data analysis, enabling another researcher to follow on with clear directives as to how the conclusions were reached. An audit trail would elaborate on how 'member checking' was done, ie. how research participants were involved in checking the emerging analysis to see if it resonated with their perspectives (Miles and Huberman, 1994). It would detail how another researcher had checked the analysis to obtain a degree of consensus on interpretation.

The use of verbatim quotes from the research participants is another common way that the authenticity of findings from interviews is verified (Polit and Hungler, 1998).

All of these processes are underpinned by researcher reflexivity: that ability of the researcher to illuminate how she/he shaped data collection and analysis through explicit acknowledgement of her/his prior beliefs and values in relation to the research area. Researcher reflexivity is central to qualitative research endeavour which seeks to be absolutely transparent about the role of the investigator in the research processes (Mauthner *et al*, 2002).

Advantages and disadvantages of semi-structured and in-depth interviews

Marchant and Kenney (2000) give a helpful list of these which summarise most of the points made so far.

Advantages

- enables the exploration of complex areas of health care
- enables a comprehensive and in-depth coverage of research area
- gives voice to patients'/clients' priorities and concerns
- enables 'on the spot' clarification of responses
- provides for flexibility around research areas
- inclusive for research participants who have problems with literacy
- achieves a high response rate.

I would add the following to this list:

- enables the meanings and interpretations of experience of patients to influence care provision
- can augment quantitative research methods and therefore gain a holistic appreciation of research topic
- gives expression to an egalitarian and partnership model of doing research between patients and healthcare professionals.

Disadvantages

- often generates huge amounts of data
- very labour intensive for the researcher
- can be expensive
- interviewer influence may lead to acceptable/orthodox responses
- generalisability often questioned due to researcher influence and small samples.

Focus groups

Focus groups have their origins in the 1980s with market research with the intent of discovering consumer preferences (Krueger, 1994). Since then health researchers have adopted it for a number of purposes. Among them:

- assessing health education messages (Basch, 1987)
- examining public understanding of illness and health behaviours (Ritchie *et al*, 1994)

- exploring the attitudes/needs of staff (Denning and Verschelden, 1993)
- developing questionnaires (Carey, 1994)
- testing more qualitatively the results of quantitative research methods (Smith, 1995).
- researching taboo subjects, for example, sexual violence (Kitzinger, 1990)
- as a consciousness-raising exercise in action research (Baker and Hinton, 1999).

This list indicates the versatility of the method and its popularity may in part be explained by the ability to assess group perspectives rapidly. However, as Kitzinger (2000) counsels, it is unwise to use the method unless the purposes of the research and the advantages of the method over, for example, individual interview, have been thought through. Some authors write of focus group's value as providing insight into the beliefs/attitudes that underlie behaviour of a specific population, examining not just what they think but how and why they think it (Carey, 1994; Asbury, 1995). Others stress the importance of the group setting and the dynamics that operate within this context for generating data of a richness and character not possible in individual interviews (Thomas *et al*, 1995).

Group work has an advantage in gaining access to different forms of communication that people use in day-to-day interaction, including jokes, anecdotes, teasing and arguing. People's knowledge and attitudes may be revealed in ways that are less likely in considered responses to direct questions as occurs in individual interviews. When group dynamics work well the co-participants act as co-researchers, taking the research in new and often unexpected directions. As Kitzinger (2000: 21) comments, 'in this sense, focus groups reach the parts that other methods cannot reach, revealing dimensions of understanding that often remain untapped by more conventional data collection techniques'.

Kitzinger (1995) suggests other advantages of focus groups over other methods:

- encourages research participants to generate and explore their own questions and to develop their own analysis of common experiences
- encourages open conversation about embarrassing subjects and permits the expression of criticism
- facilitates the expression of ideas and experiences through involvement in group debates
- helps to identify group norms/cultural values
- provides insight into the operation of group social processes in the articulation of knowledge (eg. through the examination of what information is sensitive within the group).

These last two points explain the extensive use of focus groups in cross cultural studies and work with ethnic minorities.

Groups have their own internal dynamics which can generate contrasting effects. Carey (1994) describes the censoring/conforming activity of groups when individuals, in response to their perceptions of others and others' views, adjust or withhold their contribution. He observed that negative effects predominate in group participants' data and that voicing criticisms seems to be singularly facilitated by group dynamics. Smith (1995) writes of the synergistic, bandwagon effects of groups where a particular view develops a populist momentum, influencing participants to change opinion. The synergism can result in extreme self-disclosure, the managing of which is a key role for the facilitator.

In fact, facilitating focus groups is a specialised task. She/he must set the ground rules, introduce 'ice breakers', initiate the agenda but not lead it, encourage wide participation, explore dissonance and incongruity, probe, remain neutral, attend to non-verbal behaviour, be self-aware of own beliefs/attitudes and how that may filter data, reflect summary data back to the group for their scrutiny and be sensitive to emotional affect (Morgan, 1992; Asbury, 1995). She/he may take a back seat at first but become more interventionist later, encouraging all members to contribute and even play 'devils advocate' to generate debate. Facilitators can also use props to stimulate discussion as Wilkinson (1998) did in her study of breast cancer. She passed around a breast prosthesis to be felt by participants.

Focus groups would commonly range from four to eight people and be held in a comfortable setting with refreshments available. Sitting around in a circle helps establish the right atmosphere. Sessions would normally last between one and two hours.

Observational methods

Purpose of observation

Kenney and Marchant (2000) list an impressive number of applications for observational methods of research for maternity care over recent years:

- observing verbal and non-verbal communications during labour (Kirkham, 1989)
- observation of routine clinical activities like vaginal examinations and their meaning for patients (Bergstrom et al, 1992)
- observation of environmental conditions, their affects on people's behaviour, eg. how women used bed curtains on maternity wards to maintain privacy or seek support (Burden, 1998)
- observing hierarchical staff structures on delivery suites and their effects (Hunt and Symonds, 1995).

From these examples some of the unique contributions of observational work to understanding the practice environment can be gleaned. Observation reveals the taken-for-granted assumptions and the hidden processes often not acknowledged or even recognised by those immersed within them. It aims to make the familiar strange by looking from the outside in, the so called 'etic' perspective; while at the same time capturing the experience of the insiders, the 'emic' perspective, by listening to their talk and watching their activities (Boyle, 1994). One of its key strengths is respect for the naturalistic setting and a desire not to manipulate or change this environment while observing it. It also is able to capture the known dissonance between what people say and what they do, a weakness if interviews are the sole data collection method (Deutscher, 1973).

Stages of doing observation

Negotiating access

Gaining access to the field may not be a straightforward exercise. Taylor (2001) distinguishes between the roles of 'gatekeeper' and 'sponsor'. 'Gatekeepers' are official roles that can approve or bar access to the field — essentially what clinical governance procedures for research approval consist of. 'Sponsors' describe individuals on the inside who facilitate the access of the researcher to where data collection is required and how it is done. It is the latter that may cause the most frustration for the researcher, who, after negotiating safe passage through formal approval mechanisms, may be held up by resistance in the field. Resistance manifests itself either through sponsors wanting to control access to certain areas or individuals for their own agendas or individuals refusing observation or interview. The experience of resistance and even hostility within the site can be very disabling for the research endeavour. I learnt this painful lesson when applying to research a midwifery-led unit. Despite gaining initial approval from the unit, this was withdrawn several months later after ethical approval had been obtained and the research was programmed to start. It took another six months to go through the entire process again with another research site. The importance of on-going communication with the actual site while the formal stages of approval are being negotiated cannot be overstated.

Researcher roles

The roles that a researcher takes on when doing fieldwork are classified by Rees (2003) along a continuum from full participant to complete observer. This has implications for access if the full participant role is adopted which can involve covert data collection with the identity of the researcher concealed. Rosenhan's (1973) notorious study of gaining admission to a psychiatric unit feigning mental illness rendered covert observation unethical in many researcher's eyes.

A staff member undertaking observation in his/her own clinical area, while maintaining some clinical role typifies the 'participant as observer' role. 'Observer as participant' is probably the role that most researchers adopt. Here, their primary focus is on observation but this will not preclude them from interacting with others in the setting and occasionally participating in simple tasks. 'Complete observer' is the literal 'fly-on-the-wall' observer who is present but detached. In reality, many researchers acknowledge that by their very presence, they influence and interact with the observed environment and participant observation is a more honest description of their role.

Many ethnographers refer to a 'bedding-in' period as research participants get used to the presence of the researcher. Greater openness and 'dropping one's guard' occur more often towards the end of a project as a researcher's presence becomes familiar. However, for the researcher, there needs to be an awareness about over identification or 'going native' where observer status disintegrates and a certain objectivity is lost.

The degree of reciprocity in field relationships is another issue for researchers. The observer role limits the intimacy that might naturally occur when spending extended periods of time with others. This may result in a sense of incongruity for the researcher but the overarching requirements of the study need to take precedence. Similarly, there can be tension between what participants expect of the researcher and what the researcher has decided will be their degree of participation, especially if they are similarly qualified. At the outset of the study, these expectations require clarification as far as possible.

Data collection

Observations are recorded in field notes. These can take a variety of forms from hand written notes, dictation recordings to photography or video. Examples of the type of data recorded are helpfully listed by LeCompte *et al* (1993). They answer the:

- who questions (description of the people involved, their characteristics and roles)
- what questions (what is happening, what are the rules of behaviour and variations in behaviour)
- where questions (descriptions of the physical space and layout)
- when questions (what is the timing of activities, when do conversations and interactions take place)
- why questions (goals and purposes that actors are trying to accomplish through their activities, why are there variations in behaviour).

If field notes are the backbone of recorded observations, the field journal or reflective diary records your impressions, queries, insights, feelings — in short, your reflections on what you have observed. These should be kept separate from the field notes but made contemporaneously. Good practice is to allow enough time at the end of the day or the day following fieldwork to type up both of these is an ordered way (Taylor, 2001).

There is a sense when undertaking participant observation that everything within the environment is data. Written records of various types, historical information, linked but external activities to the setting — all of these may inform the final record that will be constructed. This combination of many data sources is referred to as triangulation. The term can be misleading as researchers use it in different ways. Aside from describing multiple data collection methods, Denzin and Lincoln (2000) understand it as multiple 'lines of sight' to include different methodologies, multiple researchers and theories. Its purpose is to add depth and insight to the phenomena under study and is not primarily a check of validity. Hunt and Symonds' (1995) ethnography of a hospital delivery suite is a good example of using different data collection techniques to paint a layered picture. They used direct observation, interview and medical notes examination in explaining the problem of women being admitted too early in labour. The 'in-house' talk classified these women as 'nigglers' who exacerbated the workload without being genuine cases. Observation of interactions with these women revealed how their perspectives on their labours was re-interpreted to fit this category, and finally the medical notes recorded the diagnosis as 'false' or spurious labour. One could see that the women's actual experience was not driving midwives' care but a pre-determined diagnostic category with quite specific parameters. We know from Kirkham's (1989) work that many women are dissatisfied with this aspect of their care.

The orientation of the researcher while remaining in the field is to question the data as it is collected so that alternative explanations of phenomena are considered. Though the end point of achieving saturation with data collection is an important objective, the researcher is continually on the lookout for deviant, inconsistent data which challenges the tentative explanatory concepts so far developed. In fact, there is a sense that the data must be interrogated to peel away layers of meaning and take-for-granted assumptions, the result of which may be inconsistent and apparently irreconcilable findings. This ambivalence can often mirror life experience.

Over the period that observations are undertaken, recordings will become progressively more focused as emergent themes are distilled and followed up.

Rigour is enhanced in observations by the access to multiple data collection sources that increase 'confirmability'. Keeping an accurate audit trail is very important because of the greater complexity attached to the method.

Advantages/disadvantages of observational methods

Rees (2003) compiled the following lists of advantages and disadvantages of observational methods:

- natural setting captures with greater accuracy what actually happens as opposed to what others say happens
- 'etic' (from outside) disposition of researcher can reveal substratum patterns/ behaviours that actors in setting are unaware of
- more complex 'why' and 'how' questions in research can be explored
- multiple data collection sources enhance validity of findings.

Disadvantages of observational methods:

- actor 'reactivity' — changing behaviour while under surveillance
- researcher 'going native' and losing critical/external focus
- problems with gaining access and consent
- time-consuming and exhausting for researcher.

The use of diaries

> I've reached the point where I hardly care whether I live or die. The world will keep on turning without me and I can't do anything to change events anyway. I'll just let matters take their course and concentrate on studying and hope that everything will be all right in the end. 3 Feb, 1944

> ... but the minute I was alone I knew I was going to cry my eyes out. I slid to the floor in my nightgown and began by saying my prayers, very fervently. Then I drew my knees to my chest, lay my head on my knees and cried, all huddled up on the bare floor. A loud sob brought me back down to earth. 5 April, 1944

These are diary excerpts from a German-Jewish teenager who was forced to go into hiding with her family during the Holocaust (Frank *et al*, 2002). The statements are powerful and accurately describe pungent feelings of despair, hopelessness, desperation and desolation. In these few sentences, the reader is transported and is able to visualise and feel the situation exactly as it was.

Why use diaries in research?

The above is just one example of the depth and understanding of phenomenon and opinion that can be gained by using diaries for data collection in a research project. Anyone who has ever found an old diary that they kept as a child can confirm this, as reading it transports you back to the time and situation. You are able to imagine clearly the feelings, the people, the sounds, the smells and the memories from just a few words. This is exactly why they are useful for healthcare research, as they are able to provide the researcher with an in-depth personal perspective from that particular time point.

The following excerpt gives the reader a snapshot of the quality of the data that can be collected by using diaries. It is written in real time and thus captures the intense feelings, conflicts and difficulties that this new breastfeeding mother is experiencing:

> Most feeds last at least an hour, Rosa suckled on both breasts for at least half-an-hour and still appeared to be starving. This made me feel as if I was not doing my job properly. I was feeling so guilty, like I am not trying enough.
>
> Very tired and still very emotional.
>
> Opinions of my family and especially my mother and mother-in-law did not help. With comments like 'your milk must be too weak or even sour!' I felt that they wanted to feed her with a bottle themselves, therefore resented me feeding her. Also while I was feeding her I could not make up a tea or a meal for them.
>
> People commented all the time on how long she fed and that she was just using me as a dummy. They took away my enjoyment of breast-feeding and the feeling of satisfaction that I was giving her a good start in life. I felt that it was my private and intimate time with my baby, that built a bond between us that everyone else resented. Decided to bottle feed from now on but feeling guilty letting baby down, being a bad mum.
>
> My partner supported me to a point, but he was eager to feed her himself, which I felt like I was being selfish in the end by not letting others have the pleasure in feeding her. I need to be strong emotionally and physically to be able to cope alone (husband back at work) looking after our baby.
>
> As I did not have an adequate milk supply, I couldn't express my breast milk into a bottle as I had intended. Any milk that was there, Rosa would take and then, as she wasn't satisfied, she would not sleep long enough for my milk supply to fill up again and this began a circle that I couldn't break even when she was given a bottle. The magical bottle that was going to make her sleep! And it didn't!

Using diaries for research is an excellent way of obtaining the writer's personal perspective and experiences (diary of feelings) and/or recording events or actions (diary of events) over a period of time. A diary of feelings, for example, may be used to record women's emotions and experiences of breastfeeding (Baker *et al*, 2003), perceptions of postnatal care (MacArthur *et al*, 2002) or feelings about their partner being present at the birth of their baby (Bondas-Salonen, 1998). Diaries can also be used in a more quantitative way to monitor and record events such as menstrual pattern, feeding pattern, behaviour in babies, food intake (Mathews *et al*, 2000) and blood pressure, for example. Diaries have the advantage and the capacity to display how feelings or events may change over time. They record the experiences more or less as they happen which provides a clearer picture than relying on mental recall and reflection sometime after the event.

Diaries may be less obtrusive and intimidating than some other qualitative methods, such as interviews or observation, as they can be kept in private and the writer may be more likely to open up and express their personal feelings, although some are less able to express themselves in this way.

Diaries may be used in isolation as a single method of data collection. However, diaries may also be incorporated in a triangular approach using a variety of methods, often as a forerunner to an interview. Used in this way, the diary can help to generate questions or points that the researcher may wish to investigate further in more depth in an interview setting. Diaries may also be used as a substitute for direct observation in situations where this is not possible, such as observing neonatal behaviour in the home. A further advantage is that, unlike more obtrusive methods, the participant decides what data is recorded. This not only ensures that the emphasis is the woman's own but also means that her own behaviour, and that of others, is not altered during the process. In order to clarify these points, one can imagine a study of pregnant women's maternity experience while in prison. If the researcher observed the experience, directly or indirectly, the woman and attending wardens may behave differently and alter the experience. Diaries, however, would allow the confidential recording of the experience with no impact on external influences.

Development of a diary

Many researchers may be attracted to using diaries for data collection, as they initially appear as a way of obtaining vast amounts of data with little input or effort on the behalf of the researcher. This, however, is a huge misunderstanding, which can only lead to research that lacks rigour. As much care and preparation should be invested in the development of a diary as is given to a questionnaire or interview schedule. The format and structure of the diary must be closely considered so that pitfalls and disadvantages can be considered and/or anticipated. Every aspect of the diary should also be piloted, including guidelines and/or instructions for use, format and questions (if structured), etc. Adjustments should then be made and the whole process re-piloted until the researcher is satisfied.

If the data to be collected is longitudinal in nature, one would be naïve to expect a respondent to go away with a list of instructions and a diary and return it at a given time point and place to the researcher. This is not real world research as completion of a diary takes a lot of compliance, discipline, time and effort on behalf of the respondent. This may be one of the disadvantages of using diaries for data collection. Experience confirms that time and effort spent by the researcher making regular contact with the respondents to act as a prompt, proves worthwhile and increases compliance. This contact may be by telephone, letter or in person, whichever is the most appropriate.

On the other hand, however, many women have astounded me with the effort they have gone to, which is often driven by altruism. In a recently completed study (Lavender, 2003) women have transcribed their diaries and sent them on disc to the researcher, they have telephoned or written to inform us of change of address, sent photographs if they have been unable to explain in words and the list goes on. Many women have found taking part in a study using diaries as a method of data collection therapeutic, assisting them to gather together their feelings so that they can make their own interpretations. Some have found the diaries to be too private and confidential to share with the researchers and have thus chosen not to submit them to the project.

Diary style

The researcher must decide which format and structure would be most appropriate for the participants being studied. This will be determined by the selected theoretical approach and focus of inquiry (see *Chapters 2* and *4*). The researcher must also take into account the advantages and disadvantages of all diary styles.

Format

Once it has been decided that a diary is to be the method of choice, the world is your oyster in this age of technology as the choice has never been better. A diary is a journal of some description over a period of time. It may be in either written or verbal form in a variety of formats such as audio, video, paper or electronic. The suitability of each depends on those being studied; for example, written diaries would not be appropriate for those who are illiterate and thus verbal diaries in the form of audio or video recordings may be more appropriate. Similarly, elderly subjects may be more familiar with completing written paper diaries as opposed to operating video or audio equipment. Diaries may be useful if the respondents and the researcher speak different languages as they allow the respondent to express himself or herself freely without the interruption of an interpreter. It may be possible and/or necessary to offer the respondent a choice of which he/she may find most appropriate. There is less compliance with paper diaries than with electronic diaries in both adults with asthma (Hyland *et al*, 1993) and adults with chronic pain (Stone *et al*, 2002). It should also be recognised that respondents may fail to complete a diary, or fail to complete it on particular days or even complete it retrospectively before returning it to the researcher (Bowling, 1997). Using electronic diaries that do not allow retrospective completion would overcome this problem by improving the quality and validity of the data (Hyland *et al*, 1996).

Table 5.1 highlights briefly some advantages and disadvantages of each format.

Table 5.1: The advantages and disadvantages of various types of diary format			
Form	**Format**	**Advantages**	**Disadvantages**
Written	Paper	Easily accessible Familiar Cheap method of data collection Less intimidating May be more compliance Participants sometimes find use therapeutic Accessed anytime	Time-consuming to transcribe Writing may be difficult to read Not appropriate for illiterate Translation and transcribing may be expensive May be low compliance
	Electronic	Does not require transcription Less time-consuming for researcher May be most familiar for some respondents, eg. teenagers Can be sent directly to researcher via the internet contemporaneously therefore able accurately to assess compliance and assurance, not written in retrospect Less transcriptive errors Less time-consuming as transcription complete Retrospective entries can be barred Accurate date and time of entry can be recorded therefore data may be more accurate and valid	Not as easily accessible Equipment expensive if provided May be unfamiliar for some respondents Respondents may feel is less private and confidential May only be suitable for select groups May not be appropriate for illiterate Not accessible to those who do not have internet access or are computer illiterate
Verbal	Audio	Most common form of communication May be able to express feeling better More appropriate for illiterate Less time-consuming for respondent	More time-consuming for respondent May feel intimidated Very time-consuming to transcribe Equipment may be expensive Potential equipment failure
	Video	Additional non-verbal data May be more in-depth Able to analyse body language and context also	Participant may feel intimidated Not as easily accessible Not as familiar More time-consuming for respondent Very time-consuming to transcribe all verbal and non-verbal communication May feel less confidential Equipment may be expensive Potential equipment failure

Structure

As with questionnaires and interviews, diaries can be structured or unstructured. Unstructured are open and allow the respondent to write whatever they feel is important and in whatever form. This structure is affected the least by researcher bias as the respondent has a free reign to write/say whatever they wish without direction from the researcher. This, however, may be a disadvantage if the researcher has a more specific agenda (Robson, 2002).

The researcher must be clear from the onset what information and in what format they would like the data to be and be clear that this information is given to the writer (in either written or verbal format or both). The respondents need to know what they have to do, when, how and why. If this information is not precise, participants may have different interpretations. For example, two different participants of the same study (Lavender, 2003) wrote the following excerpts:

Anna's Diary

20th December 2000.
Baby girl born 20.21 pm. Put to breast as soon as delivered. Fed through most of the night until about 5:30 am
Next feed on 21st December 2000: 10 am and fed for about 10 minutes
12:30 pm fed for 15 minutes
4.00 pm fed for 10 minutes then fell asleep
8.00 pm fed first 20 minutes with encouragement
9:00 pm fed for 10 minutes then and 9:30 pm, 10:00 pm fed for 10 minutes each time.

22nd December 2000.
1.00 am fed for 10 minutes
3:10 am fed for 5 minutes
4:15 am fed for 10 minutes
6:05 am fed for 10 minutes
9:15 am fed for 10 minutes
12:30 pm fed for 15 minutes
3:45 pm fed for 15 minutes
A 7:45 pm fed for 10 minutes
9:00 pm fed for 15 minutes

23rd December, 2000.
1.00 am fed for 10 minutes.
5:30 am fed for 20 minutes.
9.00 am fed for 15 minutes.
11.30 am fed for 10 minutes.
2.30 pm fed for 10 minutes.

Etc. etc. etc for the rest of the diary.

Sophie's Diary

Friday 25 December

Midwife visited again and tried helping her latch on. Told me to carry on trying. It's very difficult to try her without the shield as she gets upset and doesn't take the milk properly without them. Luckily she sleeps well when visitors are here, ie. all afternoon, but night time I'm exhausted because she's awake on and off all the time.

It's impossible to catch up on sleep with all the visitors we get in the day. They don't realise we've been awake all night.

Saturday 26 December

My right nipple was bleeding and painful on the first feed. I read in my baby book (Penelope Leach *Baby and Child*) that sore cracked nipples should be rested and so decided to leave the feeding on this side.

I fed from the left side all day. Both breasts were agonisingly progressed, the right breast became very painful and engorged, and by evening the breast was leaking milk. I expressed some milk and attempted a cup feed. Camille spat most of this milk out and coughed and spluttered. By evening I was worried that she wasn't getting enough milk from the left breast as she kept wanting to be fed, and woke up a few minutes after sucking.

I felt very desperate through the night, and like I'd failed to feed my daughter. I expressed some milk — it took about 1½ hours and put it in a bottle. She took it very well and went to sleep. Although I felt that a bottle wasn't ideal I was relieved that she had settled so well after.

Sunday 27 December

In the morning I rang the midwifery service for advice and was very upset on the phone. The midwife advised me to use the right side even though it was still bleeding. She also gave some general advice, and reassurance — she arranged for an on-call midwife to come. She arrives within an hour. She was very calm and gentle and sympathetic. I felt much better after her support. She showed me how to use a slightly different position, and was very positive about everything I was doing. She helped me practice latching on without the shield, and Camille managed a few successful sucks. The most important difference was that the pain was less without the shield. Even the pain using the shield was less using the new position. (The pain was certainly wearing me down and I was beginning to dread each feed.)

I felt much more positive after this visit and wished that this midwife could have come every day.

Monday 28 December

Very tired today — more visitors. Have decided to ban visitors in the day time so that we can catch up on sleep. I'm sure that my milk supply and physical/mental condition will improve if I get more sleep. I thought Christmas would be a good time to have a baby — but it's double the stress, with the various social demands. I didn't practice the latching on enough today and just wanted her to be happy and settled.

Will make more effort tomorrow.

Night — much better sleep, although had to put her in bed with me.

It is apparent that these two respondents have different interpretations of what they were expected to do. If the researcher does not require specific information or data this is not a problem. For example, the first diary would be appropriate if the researcher was examining breastfeeding times and patterns, but not appropriate for examining in-depth feelings associated with breastfeeding, which the second diary clearly expresses. It is worth noting that if a different method of data collection had been used, ie. interviews, then the findings would have differed according to the time of inquiry. If Sophie had provided her views solely on the 26th the researcher would interpret her breastfeeding experience as negative, however, on the 27th her experience would be viewed as more positive. Extreme views and feelings are more likely to be expressed using diaries as the writer may be more compelled to record strong emotions, experiences and events.

If specific information is required then the researcher must be more explicit in the guidelines. It may be more appropriate to use a structured diary. Structured diaries may be more specific and keep the data more focused but, of course, are they open to researcher bias? The way the questions are worded may lead the respondent. Questions, as in a questionnaire may be closed or open or a combination of both and the researcher must decide which is the most appropriate. This will be dictated by the purpose of the study. In some ways, structured diaries may be more focused and easier to analyse. However, the researcher has a responsibility to ensure that the questions asked are relevant to the experience of the population being studied. Pilot work is essential to ensure the validity (Robson, 2002) of chosen questions. It is often useful to pre-print the questions within the diary at regular time points, relevant to the research. In the example below, respondents were prompted to answer the same questions at specific points in the diary — daily for the first week, weekly for a month and then monthly until completion.

Example of structured diary (Lavender *et al*, 2004)

Day 1, Week 1

What was your best experience of breastfeeding today?

What was your worst experience of breastfeeding today?

Could anyone or anything have made this experience better? If yes, please describe

Could any healthcare professional have made this better for you? If yes, please describe

---

Audit trail

Diaries are not only useful in providing the participants' perspective but they can also be extremely useful for researchers to complete. This can assist in validating the information that is written in the participant's diary and allows field notes to be recorded simultaneously. This may include environmental factors, events, researcher feelings, relevant literature and political, social and cultural influences. In a recent study (Baker *et al*, 2003) which required regular contact with respondents, I kept a personal diary, an excerpt of which can be seen below.

12 November 2001

Telephoned Beth. Husband answered and said, 'I hope she gives up this breastfeeding lark, can't you tell her to stop?' Spoke to Beth on telephone. Baby is five days old and she feels very unconfident with breastfeeding. Is in a lot of pain and doesn't feel that she will able to carry on for much longer. Has been filling in diary. Referred to Infant feeding coordinator.

22 November 2001

Telephoned Beth. She is still breastfeeding and starting to enjoy it a bit more now.

This excerpt enlightens the researcher to the possible external pressure that may be influencing the experience, ie. the husband. Beth did not actually mention this in her own diary. Furthermore, this excerpt reminds the researcher, during the analysis phase, of the conversations held with the respondent and the advice given.

Alternative approaches

In recent years, additional data collection methods have been trialed in qualitative studies.

Narrative has become increasingly popular as a way of understanding patient experience of illness. In particular, it has been used in relation to care of the elderly (Astedt *et al*, 1994), understanding mental illness (Launer, 1999) and women's experience of labour and birth (VandeVusse, 1999). Narrative is suited to exploring seminal experiences or extraordinary events in people's lives and Simkin (1992, 1990) alerted midwives to its potential as a research method in maternity care with her investigation of women's long term memories of childbirth. She found that women recalled with an amazing amount of detail events from over twenty years earlier. Narrative also contributes to an individual's integration of life events into their personal history through a process of constructing, shaping and interpreting these as they tell their story (McCance *et al*, 2001). Clouston (2003) demonstrated that a person's account can change in the retelling, revealing the layering of meaning that accumulates over time. The unstable nature of meaning-making is clearly demonstrated here and reveals the folly of trying to capture some objective evaluation of patients' experience through postal survey or structured interview. As a data collection tool it has many similarities to the in-depth interview and requires many of the same skills. The story though may be more tangential in the telling and needs to be communicated in an unstructured way to elicit nuances. Narrative is recorded and transcribed prior to analysis.

Bergstrom's *et al* (1992, 1997) widely quoted study of behaviours during the second stage of labour was conducted using video. One of the advantages of this method is the ability to capture behaviour and then replay it many times as analysis is carried out. Bergstrom demonstrated this advantage as she scrutinised the ritual of vaginal examination. Close observation of the tape led her to develop her understanding of the practice as a 'surgical' procedure, designed to neutralise the intrusiveness and inappropriateness of the entry of a sexual orifice, a practice usually reserved for the expression of intimacy and done in extreme privacy. One of the debates around the use of video has been its relative impact on the behaviours before the lens. Lomax and Casey (1998) argue that it alters natural behaviours and should be acknowledged as contributing to the forming of meaning and to the construction of knowledge in the setting where it is used. Starr (1987) disagrees, believing that research participants quickly adjust to the camera's presence. The real affect probably lies somewhere in between. In this context it is interesting to note the popularity of reality television shows in recent years, which seek successfully to make entertainment out of observing everyday behaviours of ordinary people, yet the contrived nature of the setting is plain for all to see.

More recent additions to text mediums of data collection include the internet and email and to the visual medium, photos and representational drawing. Many of these methods have become popular as researchers have struggled with the 'crisis of representation' in writing up the results of qualitative research (LeCompte, 2002). Researchers' dilemma here is to what extent their voice adequately represents their research participants in the final record. Finding alternative ways of presenting findings using a variety of mediums has been one response to this (Foley, 2002).

Final thoughts

Self-awareness and self-knowledge are important attributes for the researcher using these methods, as one's role here is not the objective, detached manager of data and indifferent recorder of findings but the reflexive, selector of data and shaper of analysis. Both are processors that require transparency and a critical disposition. The researcher is ultimately judged by the credibility of findings and their transferability to similar settings. One of the most respected exponents of these methods was instrumental in influencing maternity care policy in the 1990s and beyond with her seminal work on communication in labour (Kirkham, 1989). Her work has been frequently quoted when others write of the importance of listening to women and treating them as an individual while the institution attempts to ascribe a patient role on them. To this day, there is no better example of the relevance and 'generalisability' of these methods.

Interview, observation and diary as data collection methods are challenging, but immensely rewarding. For the researcher, they require high levels of personal commitment and discipline, exercised over many months. The often stimulating interactions of the field and the interview setting are contrasted with the many solitary hours of organising and analysing data. But these hours are fully vindicated when 'A-hah' moments result in profound insights that explain the complex or the apparently irreconcilable.

Further reading

Bourgue LB, Back KW (1982) Time sampling as a field technique. In: Burgess RG, ed, *Field Research: A Sourcebook and Field Manual*. Allen & Unwin, London: 258–59

Burgess RG (1981) Keeping a Research Diary. *Cambridge J Education* **11**: 75–83

Cluett E, Bluff R (2000) *Principles and Practice of Research in Midwifery*. Baillière Tindall, London

Coxon T (1988) Something sensational: the sexual diary as a tool for mapping detailed sexual behaviour. *Sociological Rev* **30**: 353–67

Gorin AA, Stone AA (2001) Recall biases and cognitive errors in retrospective self reports: A call for momentary assessments. In: Baum A, Revenson T, Singer J, eds. *Handbook of Health Psychology*. Erlbaum, Mahwah NJ: 405–13

Pope C, Mays N (2000) *Qualitative Research in Health Care*. BMJ Books, London

Shiffman S, Hufford M, Paty J (2001) Subject experience diaries in clinical research. Part 1: The patient experience movement. *Appl Clinical Trials* **10**: 46–56

Silverman D, ed (1997) *Qualitative Research: Theory, Method and Practice*. Sage, London

Stone AA, Turkann J, Jobe J, Bachrach C, Kurtzman H, Cain V (2000) *The Science of Self Report*. Erlbaum, Mahwah NJ

Streubert H, Carpenter D (2000) *Qualitative Research in Nursing: Advancing the Humanistic Imperative*. JB Lippincott, Philadelphia

Zimmerman DH, Wieder DL (1977) The diary: diary-interview method. *Urban Life* **5**: 479–98

References

Asbury JE (1995) Overview of focus group research. *Qualitative Health Res* **5**(4): 414–20

Astedt K, Heikinnen R (1994) Two approaches to the study of health and old age: the thematic interview and the narrative method. *J Adv Nurs* **20**(3): 418–21

Baker R, Hinton R (1999) Do focus groups facilitate meaningful participation in social research? In: Barbour R, Kitzinger J, eds. *Developing Focus Group Research: Politics, Theory and Practice*. Sage, London

Baker L, Lavender T, McFadden K (2003) Breastfeeding and family life. Current issues in Midwifery, British Journal of Midwifery Conference, Birmingham.

Basch C (1987) Focus group interview: an under-utilised research technique for improving theory and practice in health education. *Health Educ Q* **14**: 411–48

Bergstrom L, Roberts J, Skillman L, Seidel J (1992) 'You'll feel me touching you sweetie'. Vaginal Examinations during the Second Stage of Labour. *Birth* **19**(l):10–18

Bergstrom L, Seedily J, Schulman-Hull L, Roberts J (1997) 'I Gotta Push. Please let Me Push!' Social interactions during the change from first to second stage labour. *Birth* **24**(3):173–80

Bondas-Salonen T (1998) How women experience the presence of their partners at the births of their babies. *Qualitative Health Res* **8**(6): 784–800

Bowling A (1997) *Research Methods in Health: Investigating Health and Health Services*. Open University Press, UK

Boyle J (1994) Styles of ethnography. In: Morse J, ed. *Critical Issues in Qualitative Research Methods*. Sage, London: 159–85

Burden B (1998) 'Privacy or help'? The use of curtaining positioning strategies within the maternity ward environment as a means of achieving and maintaining privacy, or as a form of signaling to peers and professionals in an attempt to seek information and support. *J Adv Nurs* **27**: 15–23

Carey MA (1994) The group effect in focus groups: planning and implementing focus group research. In: Morse J, ed. *Critical Issues in Qualitative Research Methods*. Sage, London

Clouston T (2003) Narrative methods: talk, listening and representation. *Br J Occupational Therapy* **66**(4): 136–42

Danziger S (1979) On doctor watching: field work in medical settings. *Urban Life* **17**(4): 513–32

Denning JD, Verschelden C (1993) Using the focus group in assessing training needs in general practice. *Child Welfare* 72: 569–79

Denzin NK, Lincoln YS (2000) *Handbook of Qualitative Research*. Sage, London

Deutscher L (1973) *What we say/What we do: Sentiments and Acts*. Scott Formeson, Glenview

Field P, Morse J (1989) *Nursing research: the application of qualitative approaches*. Chapman & Hall, London

Foley D (2002) Critical ethnography: the reflexive turn. *Qualitative Stud Educ* **15**(5): 469–90

Frank A, Frank OH (ed), Pressler M (ed), Massatty S (translator) (2002) *Diary of a young girl*. Puffin Books, London (first published 1947)

Hammersley M, Atkinson P (1995) *Ethnography: Principles in Practice*. 2nd edn. Routledge, London

Henery N (2003) Constructions of spirituality in contempory nursing theory. *J Adv Nurs* **42**(6): 550–57

Hey V (2002) 'Not as nice as she was supposed to be': schoolgirls friendships. In: Taylor S, ed. *Ethnographic Research: A Reader*. Sage Publications, London: 67–91

Holloway I, Wheeler S (1996) *Qualitative Research for Nurses*. Blackwell Science, Oxford

Hunt S, Symonds A (1995) *The Social Meaning of Midwifery*. Macmillan, Basingstoke

Hyland ME, Kenyon CA, Allen R, Howarth P (1993) Diary keeping in asthma: comparison of written and electro methods. *Br Med J* **306**(6876): 487–89

Hyland ME, Crocker GR (1996) Diary assessments of quality of life. *Quality of Life Newsletter* **16**: 8–9

Isaia D, Parker V, Murrow E (1999) Spiritual wellbeing among older adults. *J Gerontological Nurs* **25**: 1—21

Kenney N, Marchant S (2000) Conducting observational studies. In: Proctor S, Renfrew M, ed. *Linking Research and Practice in Midwifery: A guide to evidence-based practice*. Baillière Tindall, London

Kettle C, Johanson R (2003a) Absorbable synthetic versus catgut suture material for perineal repair (Cochrane Review) In: The Cochrane Library, Issue 1, 2003a. Update Software, Oxford

Kettle C, Johanson R (2003b) Continuous versus interrupted sutures for perineal repair (Cochrane Review) In: The Cochrane Library, Issue 1, 2003b. Update Software, Oxford

Kirkham M (1989) Midwives and information-giving during labour. In: Robinson S, Thompson A, eds. *Midwives, Research & Childbirth*. Vol. 1. Chapman & Hall, London

Kitzinger J (2000) Focus groups with users and providers of health care. In: Pope C, Mays N, eds. *Qualitative Research in Health Care*. BMJ Books, London: 20–9

Kitzinger J (1990) Recalling the pain... medical procedures can bring back memories of sexual violence. *Nurs Times* **86**(3): 38–40

Kitzinger J (1995) Qualitative research: introducing focus groups. *Br Med J* **311**(1000): 299–302

Krueger R (1994) *Focus Groups: a practical guide for applied research*. Sage, London

Lavender T (2003) Breastfeeding: Expectations versus reality. The Research Findings Register (ReFer), available online at: http://www.info.doh.gov.uk

Lavender T, Thompson S, Wood L (2004) Breastfeeding guardians for teenagers: a practice based project. *Br J Midwif* (in press)

Launer J (1999) A narrative approach to mental health in general practice. *Br Med J* **318**: 117–19

Lecompte M (2002) The transformation of ethnographic practice: past and current challenges. *Qualitative Res* **2**(3): 283–99

LeCompte M, Preissle J, Tesch R (1993) *Ethnography and Qualitative Design in Educational Research*. Academic Press, Chicago

Leininger M (1985) *Qualitative Research Methods in Nursing*. Grune and Stratton, Orlando

Lomax H, Casey N (1998) Recording social life: Reflexivity and video methodology. *Sociological Research Online* **3**(2):1–31, http://www.socresonline/3/2/1.html

MacArthur C, Winter HR, Bick DE, Knowles H *et al* (2002) Effects of redesigned community postnatal care on women's health 4 months after birth: A cluster randomised controlled trial. *The Lancet* **359**(9304): 378–85

Marchant S, Kenney N (2000) Conducting interviews with individuals and groups. In: Proctor S, Renfrew M, eds. *Linking Research and Practice in Midwifery: A guide to evidence-based practice*. Baillière Tindall, London

Mathews F, Yudkin P, Smith RF, Neil A (2000) Nutrient intakes during pregnancy: the influence of smoking status and age. *J Epidemiol Community Health* **54**(1): 17

Mason J (2002) *Qualitative Researching*. Sage, London

McCance T, McKenna H, Boore J (2001) Exploring caring using narrative methodology: an analysis of the approach. *J Adv Nurs* **33**(3): 350–56

McCandlish R, Bowler U, van Asten H, Berridge G *et al* (1998) A randomised controlled trial of care of the perineum during second stage of normal labour. *Br J Obstet Gynaecol* **105**: 1262–72

Mauthner M, Birch M, Jessop J, Miller T (2002) *Ethics in Qualitative Research*. Sage, London

Maykut P, Morehouse R (1994) *Beginning Qualitative Research: A philosophic and practical guide*. The Falmer Press, London

Miles M, Huberman M (1994) *Qualitative Data Analysis: An Expanded Sourcebook*. Sage, London

Morgan DL (1992) Designing focus group research. In: Stewart M, Tudiver M, Bass E, Dunn E, Norton P, eds. *Tools for Primary Care Research*. Sage, Newbury Park: 177–94

Polit D, Hungler B (1998) *Nursing Research: Principles & Methods*. JB Lippincott, Philadelphia

Rees C (2003) *An Introduction to Research for Midwives*. Books for Midwives Press, Cheshire

Ritchie JE, Herscovitch F, Nofor JB (1994) Beliefs of blue collar workers regarding coronary risk behaviours. *Health Educ Res* **9**: 95–103

Rosenhan D (1973) On being sane in insane places. *Science* **179**: 250–8

Robson C (2002) *Real World Research*. 2nd edn. Blackwell Publishers Ltd, Oxford

Sackett D, Rosenberg W, Gray J, Haynes R (1996) Evidence-based medicine: what it is and what it isn't. *Br Med J* **312**: 71–2

Salmon D (1999) A feminist analysis of women's experiences of perineal trauma in the immediate post-delivery period. *Midwifery* **15**(4): 247–56

Simkin P (1992) Just another day in a woman's life? Part 2: Nature and consistency of women's long-term memories of their first birth experiences. *Birth* **19**(2): 64–81

Simkin P (1990) Just another day in a woman's life? Women's long-term perceptions of their first birth experiences. Part 1. *Birth* **18**(4): 203–10

Smith MW (1995) Ethics in focus groups: a few concerns. *Qualitative Health Res* **5**(4): 478–86

Starr R (1987) Clinical judgements of abuse-proness based on parent-child interactions. *Child Abuse Neglect* **11**: 87–92

Stone AA, Shiffman S, Schwartz JE, Broderick JE, Hufford MR (2002) Patient non-compliance with paper diaries. *Br Med J* **324**(7347): 1193–94

Taylor S (2001) *Ethnography: Master Programme Module D844*. Open University Press, London

Thomas L, MacMilllan J, McColl E, Hale C, Bond S (1995) Comparison of focus group and individual interview methodology in examining patient satisfaction in nursing care. *Soc Sci Health* **1**(4):206-20

VandeVusse L (1999) Decision making in analyses of women's birth stories. *Birth* **26**(1): 43–50

Van Teijlingen E, Ireland J (2003) Research interviews in midwifery. *RCM Midwives* **6**(6): 260–62

Walsh D (1999) An ethnographic study of women's experience of partnership caseload midwifery practice: the professional as friend. *Midwifery* **15**(3): 165–76

Wilkinson S (1998) Focus groups in health research. *J Health Psychol* **3**: 323–42

Chapter 6

How do you analyse qualitative data?

Bernie Carter

I have yet to see any problem, however complicated, which when you looked at it in the right way, did not become still more complicated.

Poul Anderson, as cited in Barrow, 1991

Introduction

The chapter title 'How do you analyse qualitative data?' is seductive. It suggests that there should be a relatively easy answer and that by the end of the chapter you should be fully prepared, confidently and competently, to undertake the analysis of your data. However, the very nature of qualitative data and qualitative data analysis means that this is unlikely. One of the few points of consensus in qualitative analysis is how difficult it is to explain 'how to do it', since producing a step-by-step recipe of 'how to do analysis' ultimately destroys the creativity and flexibility inherent in the analytical process. In many research texts, analytical processes are alluded to (Clarke, 1999) and very abstract terms are used. While I do not believe that these are intentionally used to mystify the process, they do not shed light on what a novice researcher needs to do.

Within this chapter I will present a number of principles and suggestions, some drawn from the literature, others from my own experiences of doing data analysis and some from helping to guide students through the confusing landscape of data analysis. This chapter will, necessarily, act as a jumping off point for further reading and further exploration of the primary texts and for deeper thinking about your own data. The tension for any qualitative researcher writing a chapter on 'how to do analysis' is that clarifying concepts, processes and issues often means that they become very over-simplified. They become easy to follow but are basically meaningless. So, with this in mind, the following chapter attempts to whet your appetite, stimulate your imagination and avoid the following situation.

Student: (on the phone) *Hi, Bernie. It's me. I know it's been a while but can I come and see you? I've got a bit of a problem. I'm stuck and running out of time. I've got all my interviews now and I've transcribed them all … I think… (although I'm not so sure now that I've done this right)… … And like… well now…. now all I need to do is get the analysis over and done with. And then I can write it up and submit.*

Bernie: *Hallo… Nice to hear from you… So what you want to talk about?*

Student: *Well… … I've got a huge pile of interview transcripts and…. and to be honest, I have no clue what to do. I've read them through but there's so much of it and I … so any ideas of what I do next? I've actually been wishing I'd done a quantitative study instead!*

(At this point the student's own sense of impending doom is generously shared with their supervisor!)

What do we mean by qualitative data?

The type of data you have collected will, of course, affect the way that you analyse them. Data can come from many different sources including interviews, focus groups, diaries, observation, stories, field notes, visual sources (such as graffiti, films, photographs, drawings) and many others. What is important to realise is that qualitative data are not inert. Your data are dynamic and changing. Your transcript(s) are not your data; they are representations or constructions of the data. Your data are your primary source materials — the interviews or focus groups, the photographs or diaries, your observations and your experiences in the field. As such, you need to appreciate that you will have already been analysing the data (even if this has been implicit and unconscious, rather than explicit and conscious) long before you might sit down to 'do your analysis'. Every decision that you take about your research has an impact on the data. Each decision has involved some level of analysis and will have shaped what you can do with your data.

What is data analysis and what are the key processes?

Analysis is not simply a matter of classifying, categorising, coding, or collating data. Most fundamentally, analysis is about the representation or reconstruction of social phenomena. We do not simply 'collect' data; we fashion them out of our transactions with other men and women. Likewise, we do not merely report what we find; we create accounts of social life and, in doing so, we construct versions of the social worlds and social actors that we observe. It is, therefore, inescapable that analysis implies 'representation' (Coffey and Atkinson, 1996: 108)

Qualitative data analysis does not attempt to present reality: it is interpretative (hermeneutic). Qualitative analysis is based within post-modernism and accepts that there will be both a multiplicity of voices heard and a multiplicity of ways in which they could be represented (Cheek, 1999). In other words, different researchers will perceive and interpret data in different ways. However, this does not mean that what is produced is dismissible and meaningless and lacks credibility. Indeed, scholarly and disciplined qualitative data analysis is full of meaning and difficult to dismiss.

Being iterative and reflexive

Analysis of qualitative data is not something that you do to your data, analysis is a cyclical, reflective process that you do **with** your data (in the same way that you don't do qualitative research **on** subjects but **with** participants). Qualitative data analysis is an ongoing process through all stages of the research and it is iterative. This means that data analysis is something that you repeatedly return to and reconsider and are reflexive about. Reflexivity involves you in subjecting yourself to critical self-scrutiny (but not 'excruciating self-confession') (Seale, 1999) considering your influence on your data. As Mason (1996: 6) states: '… the very art of posing difficult questions to oneself in the research process is part of the activity of reflexivity.' As you revisit your data you will question whether you need more or different data, whether or not you need to interrogate your data in a new way. This helps you to build up layers of analysis and re-analysis. Analysis is likely to be complex and it often feels messy. It is not something you can 'get over and done with quickly'.

Three key (but not linear) processes

There are many different suggestions or definitions about data analysis, with different writers proposing different terminology to describe the principles. However, almost all definitions would encompass the notion that data (interviews, observations, etc) need to be prepared for systematic, rigorous analysis through the process of transcription (turning words, images, notes, etc into text). The data then needs to be read actively. Three other major processes follow:

⌘ Data reduction (breaking data down and decontextualising data). The 'process of selecting, focusing, simplifying, abstracting, and transforming the data' (Miles and Huberman, 1994: 10).

⌘ Data display (bridges between reduction and complication) and refers to 'an organised, compressed assembly of information that permits conclusion drawing and verification' (Miles and Huberman, 1994: 10).

⌘ Data complication (involves conclusion drawing through building data up and reintegrating context, and verification of data) (Huberman and Miles, 1994: 429).

In an almost blasphemous attempt to present an iterative, dynamic, reflexive, comparative, cyclical process in an (over) simplified manner, the following diagram (*Figure 6.1*) presents in a linear form an overview of the process.

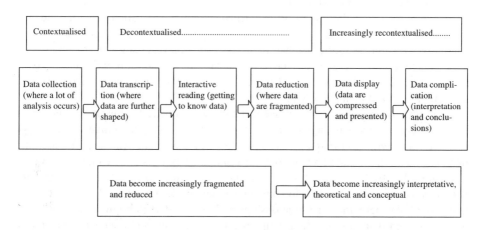

Figure 6.1: A simplified and linear representation of the processes within data analysis

However, you cannot simply think of these processes as stages that you can follow in a linear and chronological manner. You cannot, for instance, plan your research week by saying: 'OK, Monday — interview, Tuesday — transcription, Wednesday — active reading, Thursday — data reduction, Friday — data display, Saturday — data complication. Analysis is finished! Sunday — write up.' You need to stay true to the notion of being iterative. At any one time you may be examining a piece of text and reducing your data using line-by-line coding, while at the same time seeing links with previous codes and making notes of these (data display) and starting to speculate abstractly about the meaning of the data (data complication). For some people this seems to be a recipe for chaos, and in some ways it is. But qualitative analysis is a form of disciplined and scholarly handling of chaos (and this is one of the reasons why your field notes are so important). Field notes can constitute a record of your ideas, impressions, feelings, observations about your research study. Field notes do not just get made when you are in the field (for example, when you are out in the clinic interviewing women or running the focus group of expectant dads): the field extends to all your own thinking about the study. The dedicated researcher carries pen and paper, or dictaphone, or post-it notes or whatever with them wherever they go, so they can note new thoughts about codes, links, relationships, concepts, gaps, etc. Your field notes become an important analysis decision audit trail, allowing you to return to the rationale for a particular code some months further on in your study.

A better, although messy, illustration of what you might be doing during data analysis can be seen in the following diagram (*Figure 6.2*). Again, it remains far too linear and two-dimensional to genuinely represent what happens. In reality there would be many more lines crossing and re-crossing. Additionally, you are not undertaking your analysis in a vacuum. Ideas, triggers and concepts will come from both within your data and from outside your data. Conversations with colleagues, academic (and casual) reading, questions from participants and ideas from the media can stimulate new ways of thinking about and with your data.

Having seen that data analysis is intrinsically messy, challenging (and hugely enjoyable) it is not surprising that things can go wrong. Many potentially good qualitative researchers fail to achieve their goal since they get stuck in the process of data reduction. Other researchers move into data complication too early and develop naive, unsubstantiated concepts and theories because they have devoted insufficient time and thought to data reduction.

The notion of reducing data may seem at odds with a qualitative research philosophy since, surely, reductionist approaches are undertaken by quantitative researchers? However, data reduction in qualitative research is necessary as without it you are left, like the student in the earlier scenario, with a pile of transcripts and no clue as to where to go next. The trick (or the scholarly and academic discipline, whichever you prefer) with data reduction is not to lose too much information. Data display allows you to start to explore links, networks, and relationships within your data through the use of visual display. Within data complication, you search for meaning and conclusions and you move from the fragmented, coded data to more conceptual and theoretical findings.

While the process is cyclical, each element is dependent upon the quality and soundness of judgment of previous elements. If the data you have collected are inadequate, for example, because of poor interviewing skills, your transcriptions will be constructions of that inadequate data and you will find it difficult to go much beyond data reduction. Good quality data does not necessarily mean reams of paper sitting on your desk or hundreds of interviews. Indeed, someone with three in-depth interviews could have better data than someone who has superficially and inconsistently interviewed say thirty or three hundred people.

What way(s) should I use to analyse my data?

Probably the most important thing to remember about qualitative data analysis is that there is no single right or wrong way to analyse data (although some could be more right than others, in particular, circumstances). For most researchers working within health care, the time to choose your approach to data analysis is when you are writing your proposal and establishing your research design. It is vital for your analytical approach to be clearly identified and substantiated, as this aspect of your proposal will be scrutinised by Scientific and Research Committees and Research Ethics Committees. Qualitative research is organic and somewhat unpredictable, but it does need to be rigorous, well-planned and executed; 'stuff might happen' but it needs to happen rigorously! It also needs to be transparent.

Novice researchers often utilise thematic analysis as their chosen analytical approach. Perhaps this is because it is apparently easier for people to get to grips with the concepts underpinning it and the language used to explain it. Broadly, thematic analysis is an approach that draws codes into groups, the groups into sub-themes, the sub-themes into themes and then the themes into a global theme that pulls everything together (see Attride-Stirling, 2001 for a particularly clear description). Although thematic analysis is relatively easy to start to work with, it requires just as much care and attention as the other, seemingly more complex approaches. All qualitative data analysis requires a researcher to be thorough, sensitive to the data, scholarly and to take care with the data.

It is beyond the scope of this chapter to present, discuss and demonstrate 'how to do' analysis within all of the differing approaches. However, the principles that follow provide a basic insight into the sorts of issues, challenges, decisions, joys and catastrophes that await any qualitative researcher.

How do you transcribe your data?

Maybe the first question that should be asked is: 'why should you transcribe your data?'

Student: (by email) *Bernie, I was also thinking re the transcribing plan I had — would it be OK just to listen and relisten and relisten to the tapes rather than transcribing them? I'm going to get swamped with tapes and work's really busy. Finding someone to do it or doing it myself would take up too much time. What do you think?*

Bernie: (short answer) *No.*

(A longer and more detailed rationale followed.)

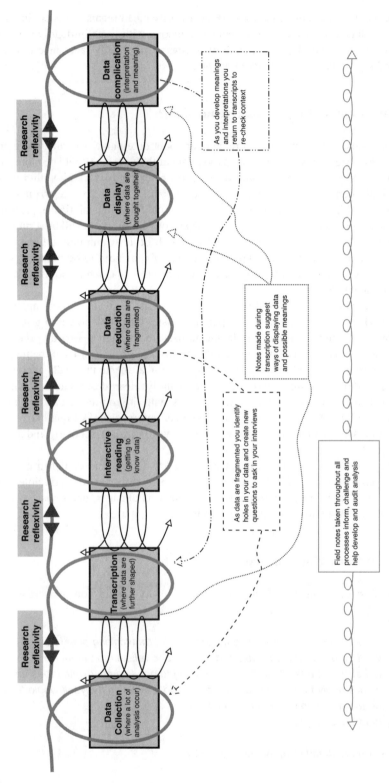

Figure 6.2: A more realistic, although still two-dimensional, representation of data analysis. (Note: a few examples illustrate this figure to show the ways in which you move back and forth through the complex process of analysis)

It is important to understand why such a time-consuming process is so vital. The temptation is that listening to tapes can circumvent transcription. However, you can never really get to know your data in the same way. It's almost impossible to juggle with data that is only in your head in the same way that you can when it's both on paper and in your head. At its most basic, transcription 'preserves data' making it more 'permanent, retrievable, examinable and flexible' (Lapadat, 2000: 204). The transcripts are the materials, along with the original written, graphic, spoken data, that you work on during the process of moving through data reduction to data complication. Just as (you might expect by now) there is no right or wrong way to analyse your data, there is no one right way to transcribe. The decisions about what and how you transcribe are ultimately dependent on the aim(s) and intent of your analysis and study. Often transcription is seen to be unproblematic, but this oversimplifies something that dramatically shapes the material you subsequently work with.

While it is impossible to transcribe everything from a research encounter (for example, every word, pause, emphasis, intonation, gesture, nuance, context, feeling, etc), it is important to attempt to transcribe the encounter in sufficient detail for you to be able to undertake appropriate and competent analysis. As a general rule, it is better to transcribe more detail than less, providing you know why the detail is likely to be useful (and to whom it will be useful). For example, a closely annotated transcript may be extremely important for a researcher interested in the way that language is used (for example, in a specific approach such as discourse analysis) but such detail may make it completely incomprehensible to non-experts reading the transcripts. If your study involves member checking, you will need to have transcripts that can be easily read by your participants. Member checking involves returning the transcripts (and sometimes other materials) to the individual participants so that they can add, delete, and clarify issues. Member checking means that your data continues to develop after the original data were collected. Member checking can be used to confirm the interpretation of the researchers. While some researchers lay great faith in member checking as a means of enhancing the credibility of their study, Meadows and Morse (2001) argue that ensuring credibility is the responsibility of the research team.

There are a number of transcription conventions (ways of transcribing) and these can be extremely important as they help to ensure that transcription within your study is consistent. Conventions include the way you lay your page out, how much detail you transcribe in terms of every word spoken, pauses in speech (eg. do you count the number of seconds and note this?), intonation, dialect, turn taking, laughs, crying, inaudible segments, segments you are not sure you have heard accurately, context, your feelings and responses and so on. The list of what you could legitimately transcribe is almost endless but you have to make those decisions. Ultimately, the material you will analyse will reflect those decisions.

Unless you are looking specifically at the linguistic construction of the text, many researchers will transcribe data in a form that looks a little like the script of a play. Line numbering allows you more easily to find specific data segments, quotes or parts of the text. Providing a wide right margin gives you room to make margin notes and insert codes. Pseudonyms will need to be used and anonymity and confidentiality ensured in both the paper and electronic copies of the transcripts. You need password protected files and a coding system to assign either pseudonyms (eg. Amy = first participant, Betty = second, Carrie = third, and so on) or numbers (eg. P1, P2, P3 [participant 1] etc).

1 Bernie. So... please can you tell me about
2 what you felt when you first started to try breast-feeding your baby?
3 Amy. [*Amy is cradling her baby.*] Well... it
4 was kind of amazingly scary and **really** beautiful
5 [*looks at baby and smiles*]... but mostly kinda
6 scary. The like, the midwives had said how to
7 do things... it and I'd been to all the classes and
8 read all the books and talk to loads of people...
9 ... But... when it came to the crunch and
10 even though the midwife is there I thought
11 you... 'Well little boy. It's just you and me and
12 we're gonna get it right. I've not done this
13 before, s:::::::o... you're gonna have to help me
14 out' [*looks at baby again and hugs him tighter*].
15 And he kind of looked at me and I knew we
16 could do it... ... MAGIC! ... ... even though it's
17 been a bit like a tightrope walking without a safety net at times.

Even if using a fairly direct and simple form of transcription you will have to make decisions about punctuation. How do you know where to place the commas, where to end sentences and where you start new paragraphs? All of these decisions, however minor they might seem, will influence the material you subsequently data reduce and then complicate. Punctuation should respect the rhythm and pace of the verbal speech and not be used to 'sanitise' the text. There are established transcription conventions (*Table 6.1*, adapted from Silverman 1993: 118) that you can use.

The level of detail used and the conventions that you use are, to a degree, up to you and the intent of your research. Providing you keep a record of what conventions you're using for a particular study (in your field notes) you can devise your own, for example ... (is a short pause), ... (is a longer pause). Other challenges you face are transcribing dialect, colloquialisms, laughter and some of the paralanguage such as grunts, groans and body language (for example, shaking head, looking surprised, smiling) and so on. All of these are much more complex to transcribe than you might first think.

Transcription is laborious and time-consuming, regardless of your typing speed. Some people transcribe first by hand and transfer handwritten notes to the computer, while others transcribe directly to the computer, and other people use voice-activated software (although this is by no means the complete labour-saving device it is made out to be). Despite the time transcription takes it does help you get close to (or extremely familiar with) your data. Some researchers will ask other people (research assistants, transcribers, family friends) to transcribe their data. This does reduce some of the potential for getting close to your data but often it may be the only realistic way of turning tapes into text. However, even though a competent typist may have entered the data onto the word processor you, as the researcher, **must** check the text file against the original audiotape, videotape, diary, or field note, etc. You will need to apply yourself to ensuring that the data is presented as appropriately as it can be within the construct of the transcript. It is also important for you to ensure that your transcriber fully understands the need for maintaining the security, confidentiality and anonymity of your original data and the transcripts. Careful procedures should be used to ensure copies are not mislaid or retained. Good practice would require that the transcriber sign a statement assuring confidentiality and a commitment to working within the Data Protection Act.

Table 6.1: Frequently used transcription conventions (adapted from Silverman, 1993)	
(.)	Indicates a tiny gap in speech
(.3)	Indicates elapsed time in silence in tenths of a second
Really	Underscoring indicates some form of stress by amplitude or pitch
( )	empty parentheses indicate that the transcriber couldn't hear the words to transcribe
MAGIC!	words in upper case denote loud sounds relative to surrounding talk
S::o	indicates the prolongation of the immediately prior sound
S:::::o	more colons indicate the length of prolongation

How do you read your data?

Many of us take reading for granted and just do it, but close, careful and iterative reading of your data is an important part of the data analysis. Simply passively reading the words is insufficient; you need to be active and you almost need to interview your data. You can simply ask five very basic questions — how, what, where, when, and why? Alternatively, you can start to ask more complex questions, such as: 'do I understand what is going on here?' 'what is being said (or not said) here?', 'do I need to check this again with the audio tape/ diary?', 'what should I have asked to find out more about this?', 'what's surprising me about my data?'. This close and comprehensive reading and re-reading lays the foundations for the next part of the process: data reduction. There are many different types of structured techniques that can be used to make your reading interactive. Dey (1993) provides a good overview of these and in which situations they might be most relevant.

How do you code and display your data?

Coding is not analysis. It is part, albeit an important part, of the whole process of analysis. The term coding is contested and the term is open to different interpretations. However, most researchers would agree that, at its most basic, coding is a way of organising data. But, if coding only operates at the level of labelling and organising data, it does not really tell you anything more about the data at all. All it allows you to do is to put everything assigned the same code in the same place. To take coding from a mere labelling exercise and to move it into a more analytical approach, the researcher and the data need more strongly to interact with each other. The researcher needs to work with the data in a more conceptual way, asking questions, such as: 'what is going on here?' 'what do I understand about this data?', 'how does this relate to other instances?' In this way, a researcher makes the data problematic. In the context of qualitative analysis, problematic is good as it means you are seeing beyond the obvious and into your data's inherent complexity.

Data reduction

There are two main starting points for coding. The first one is where you approach your data with a set of already established (*a priori*) codes that you have generated from the literature, from your own thinking about your research, and from any theoretical or conceptual frameworks that you have drawn on or utilised in your study. This approach can be helpful but it can limit your analysis. If you simply stick with the *a priori* codes and you do not add to, amend, or discard codes your analysis is likely to suffer from being static and unresponsive to your discoveries. The second approach is much more inductive, and aligned to Strauss's notion of *in-vivo* coding, whereby the codes that you assign arise from the words, ideas and concepts that your participants are using (for example, you may chose to stay very close to the participants' language by using the word 'scary' rather than, say, 'fearful' as your code name). Using an inductive approach helps you to stay close to your data and to work in a way that is more likely to be recognised by your participants. Regardless of whether you are working with *a priori* or *in-vivo* codes or with a mixture of both, clarity about coding is essential. It is important that you note (define) what you mean by each code you assign (for example, the code 'fear' may be defined by you in the context of your study as '… relating to words that suggest that that the mothers are worried, frightened, anxious or scared'). This means that you start to compile your code list as part of the field notes as you go along. This is particularly important if you are undertaking analysis over a period of time. It is sometimes easy to forget what you actually meant by a code when you come back to analysis some time later.

Coding is a dynamic process. As you start to work more closely with your data and develop greater and greater insight you will need to abandon some codes that seemed sensible or important but which have outlived their usefulness. Other codes will need to be changed, for example, the wording changed or tightened to reflect your enhanced understanding. New codes will be created as you suddenly see something in your data that you missed on a previous run-through. As you make these changes you need to ensure that a code that is changed in transcript six, for example, is modified throughout the rest of the transcripts. A code that is created during your analysis of a later transcript will need to be looked for in all the previous transcripts. All of this is labour-intensive work and requires you to be thorough in your cycles of reading and re-reading the texts. No one gets coding right first time. Often when you look back at your first run-through of coding you will see that you were quite naive, superficial and missed many things out. It can be quite daunting starting to code, but you have to start somewhere. Possibly the easiest practical way to start is to mark the transcript with coloured highlighter pens and to make margin marks with tentative code labels. At this stage, people often under-code (hardly code anything or code huge sweeps of text with one code) or they over-code (virtually everything is coded with no real rationale). These, to some extent, reflect the uncertainties of the novice coder but they also reflect the two extremities of coding.

Very inclusive codes can be useful to give you an indication of the main issues, but they give little indication of the subtleties that are inherent in your data. It is those subtleties, nuances and interpretations that are vital if you are to start getting involved with, learning from and understanding the meanings within your data. However, this first naïve trawl is almost inevitable as even the most expert and experienced researcher has to start somewhere.

For example — some fairly inclusive codes:

1	Bernie. So... please can you tell me about	
2	what you felt when you first started to try	
	breast-feeding your baby?	
3	Amy. [*Amy is cradling her baby*] Well... it	
4	was kind of amazingly scary and <u>really</u> beautiful	
5	[*looks at baby and smiles*]... but mostly kinda	'scary'
6	scary. The like, the midwives had said how to	
7	do things... it and I'd been to all the classes and	'preparation'
8	read all the books and talk to loads of people...	
9	... But... ... when it came to the crunch and	
10	even though the midwife is there I thought	
11	you... 'Well little boy. It's just you and me and	
12	we're gonna get it right. I've not done this	
13	before, s::::o ... you're gonna have to help me	'mother and baby team'
14	out' [*looks at baby again and hugs him tighter*].	
15	And he kind of looked at me and I knew we	
16	could do it... ... MAGIC! ... ... even though it's	
17	been a bit like a tightrope walking without a safety net at times.	

For example – some more detailed codes:

1	Bernie. So... please can you tell me about	
2	what you felt when you first started to try	
	breast-feeding her baby?	
3	Amy. [Amy is cradling her baby] Well... it	'Scary' 'really beautiful'
4	was kind of amazingly scary and really beautiful	(emotional responsive-
		ness 'scary' (but not quite)
5	[*looks at baby and smiles*]... but mostly kinda	'professionals/midwives' 'how to
6	scary. The like, the midwives had said how to	do' 'preparation/classes'
7	do things ... it and I'd been to all the classes and	'prepartion/books' 'preparation/
8	read all the books and talk to loads of people...	people' 'crunch time' 'midwife/
9	... But ... ... when it came to the crunch and even	support' 'just you and me'
10	though the midwife is there I thought you... 'Well	'get it right' 'not prepared' 'help
11	little boy. It's just you and me and we're gonna get	me out' 'baby-reassures' baby
12	it right. I've not done this before, s::::o you're	behaviour/look 'can do it'
13	gonna have to help me out' [*looks at baby again*	'magic' 'scary' 'tightrope' 'safety
14	*and hugs him tighter*]. And he kind of looked at	net' (ongoing experience)
15	And he kind of looked at me and I knew we could	(maybe liminality)
16	do it... ... MAGIC! ... ... even though it's been a	
17	like tightrope walking without a safety net at times.	

Whilst both of the above examples demonstrate coding, they don't really demonstrate analysis. They don't show what is really going on or what is behind the dialogue we can see in the transcript. They have labelled the data but not helped to explain it.

Data coding and the analytical processes that accompany it involve being cyclical and returning and returning to the text. As you do this you gradually develop more insightful codings and interpretations and a greater awareness of what has been said and what has been omitted. As you go deeper into and get closer to your data you gradually develop an assuredness based on your own reflexive stance. Returning to your data helps to determine if it bears out the concepts and theories that are beginning to emerge from the time spent being with and thinking with your data. Savage (2000) talks of the spaces in data where things that are not said appear as important as the things that are said. In interviews, people may describe the out of the ordinary even though the 'ordinary is there in the background'.

For those researchers more used to working with quantitative data this move away from simply 'labelling coding' to 'interpretation coding' can be fraught. It is at this point, perhaps more than any other, when the analysis moves beyond mere facts. If we take just one line from the previous example: 'Well... it was kind of amazingly scary and really beautiful... but mostly kinda scary'. Simple label coding could result in fairly mechanistic codes being applied such as, 'scary' or 'fear' or 'anxiety' or as 'scary – mother.' Deeper coding would attempt to organise deeper issues and interpretations such as 'balance of extreme emotions', 'beauty overwhelming fear', 'powerful first impressions' and so on. Throughout all three processes (reduction, display and complication) you will be using comparison as a means of helping to clarify your understanding. You will be comparing your data with the findings from other studies as well as comparing the findings that start to emerge with what you perhaps expected. Comparison, at all levels, is a dominant principle underpinning qualitative research (Boeije, 2002).

Data display

Regardless of whether the coding is fairly naive or becoming conceptually more sophisticated (and often more theoretical at the same time) there is a need for the researcher to be able to organise, compress, access and visually explore their codes through data display (Miles and Huberman, 1994). There are many different approaches to exploring and displaying your data. Broadly speaking, people structure their data in ways that suit themselves and their own particular ways of working and thinking. Some people prefer maps or diagrams, others use matrices, index cards, post-it notes or computer supported retrieval programmes to help them develop a system to explore their data in as many different ways as possible. One of the principles underpinning this part of the process is flexibility. The researcher will often start by putting all data segments or fragments that have the same code name (eg. all the data segments that have been assigned the code 'scary' from all the interviews) into the same place (see *Table 6.2*). This might be in a Word file, or more simply listed on a piece of paper titled 'scary' with note of the originating transcript and line number (for example, Amy line 4 might be presented as A,l4).

You then literally start to play, albeit a scholarly form of playing, by putting codes that relate to and have a sense of belonging to each other together. Codes that belong to a group, by implication, do not usually belong to another group. Grouping codes involves differentiating between what is included and what is excluded. This, in itself, can help you develop better insight and understanding of your data. Groups need to be meaningful, both in relation to your data and the other groups you are developing (Dey, 1993: 96–97). You might put all the codes relating to emotions and feelings (for example, scary, elated, amazed, full of love, happy) together or you might put codes relating to mother and baby as a team together ('you and me', 'we're a team' 'we'll help each other'). The act of scholarly playing means that you start to see what happens when you bring different codes together into a group (sometimes called a code family or a theme). Just as you started coding in a quite naïve way, you may find that you start to draw the codes together in a fairly unsophisticated way as well. Again, as you start to appreciate your data in deeper ways you will start to perceive that other groupings are possible and, indeed, allow you to develop stronger groupings and meanings. You may find at this stage that some of your coding is not working and you need to go back and re-code your data, or you need to look for and code for issues that you have just become aware of while you have been undertaking data display.

Table 6.2: Example of data fragments belonging to the code 'scary'
Code: 'scary'
it was kind of amazingly scary (A, 14) but mostly kinda scary (A, 15) a bit like a tightrope walking without a safety net at times (A, 115–17) I was a bit freaked out at first (j, 13) It was worrying really (H, 112) Scared in a way (D, 19)

Researchers can become frustrated as they are left with some codes that do not fit the pattern that is beginning to emerge from their data display. Do not ignore these. These are just as important as the codes that fit, as these outside codes/themes/families can help you to construct more insightful questions to ask your data. This eventually helps you to a deeper understanding of your data. Things that do not fit can help you pose additional questions to participants. Life itself does not fit readily into completely ordered patterns and boxes and neither do data from qualitative studies.

Figure 6.3 is a simple example of how relationships can be mapped. Other, more complex, visual displays can be used to illustrate other relationships, connections and networks. For example, you might want to track the journey that each participant travelled (*Figure 6.4*), where the use of different symbols/shading can help you see relationships more clearly. Using different emphasis in the lines can reflect the strength or importance of particular issues or concepts.

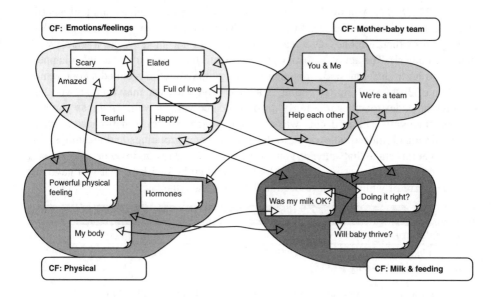

Figure 6.3: An example of data display (drawing on four code families, codes have been placed in code families (CF) and some links between families have been established)

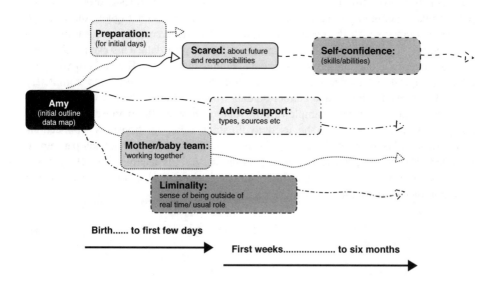

Figure 6.4: Example of visual display of data over time

Data complication

Data complication requires you to draw upon your inferential skills as you 'dig deeper'(Froggatt, 2001a). Digging deeper involves considering new frames of reference and dimensions and identifying and following new lines of speculation. Creative thinking and the formation of tentative hypotheses about your data accompany the process of speculation. Speculation can feel precarious and uncertain. It's a bit like playing a game where you don't know the rules. However, as you get to know your data better and better, you gradually create the rules and start to feel increasingly secure. Data complication occurs as you move deeper through cycles of coding, display and reflexivity until you eventually get to a point where the relationships between and within codes and themes are firmly established and understood. You generate a sense of things belonging to each other and you can move towards the theory building. Patterns start to develop, and the groupings and relationships that you have created strengthen and develop internal coherence and have resonance with your research questions and within the context of your study.

You may be lucky to have a 'Eureka!' moment (a moment when the 'pattern' becomes fully established and has meaning for you). It is almost impossible for this aspect of data analysis to be reduced to a 'how to do it recipe'. This is because only you, as the researcher, can make this happen through your intense and close association with your data. Outsiders (colleagues, supervisors, and critical friends) may be able to make suggestions, such as: 'Have you thought of considering the concept of "x" (eg. risk) as a way of making sense of your data?' or 'I think that you might find reading about "y" (eg. catastrophe theory) helpful'. But only you can know if such suggestions are helpful or relevant. At times, someone will make a suggestion that, almost immediately, you know is wrong or doesn't fit your data. Don't ignore it, as it may help to clarify issues and bring you nearer to knowing what sort of explanatory framework or theory does fit your data. Using metaphor as a thinking tool can also help you to interpret your findings (Aubusson, 2002).

While there are no hard and fast rules as to how you complicate or confront your data, Dey (1993: 227) proposes that there are five different procedures for encouraging you to confront your data:

- ❖ 'enumerate the amount of data
- ❖ evaluate the quality of evidence
- ❖ assess the conceptual significance of the d ata
- ❖ look for exceptions, extreme or negative examples
- ❖ follow different pathways through the data.'

One way of appreciating the Eureka moment is to imagine you're looking through a child's kaleidoscope, turning the end and seeing lots of different patterns made out of the fragments of crystal (codes in this case). Each turn creates a pattern that is quite pleasing and patterns you are reasonably happy with. However, you continue turning and then, suddenly, the pattern presented is the one that you like the best because of the ways that colours relate to each other and the pattern (for you) has fallen into perfect place. This gives you some sort of a feel for what you will experience when your data kaleidoscope reveals the pattern of your findings. The revealed pattern then needs to be systematically and rigorously checked to determine that it does genuinely arise from and can be substantiated by your data (even when it has moved beyond it). This involves more thinking **with** your data and being reflexive.

Data complication involves the generation of new ideas that arise from the data. These new ideas and concepts allow you to start to create novel ways of explaining what you have discovered. This process requires you to continue to be open-minded about what you think you have discovered; about what you think your findings are. As you start to uncover and discover new ideas and meanings from your data you need to check that they are substantiated by your data and that they are new. While it is almost impossible to come up with a genuinely new idea, it is possible to come up with a new twist on an existing idea or to transfer an idea or concept from one discipline into another. As Coffey and Atkinson (1996: 158) state:

> *Our task as qualitative researchers is to use ideas in order to develop*
> *interpretations that go beyond the limits of our own data and that go beyond*
> *how previous scholars used that. It is in that synthesis that new interpretations*
> *and new ideas emerge. The point is not to follow previous scholarship*
> *slavishly but to adapt and transform it in the interpretation of one's own data.*

It is all too easy to start to feel overwhelmed by the prospect of developing a theory; it can seem like an almost unachievable task. However, a theory is broadly a set of ideas about an issue that help explain it. If we think of theory in these terms, contributing to theory development or proposing a theory as a result of our research becomes more achievable. Dey (1993: 51) debunks some of the stuffiness associated with theory when he proposes theory:

> *... simply as an idea of how other ideas can be related.......... [theory can]*
> *provide the necessary direction and organizing framework through which to*
> *bring together the different concepts used in our analysis.*

Until you have swum in the depths of the shark-infested custard of your own data, it is difficult for a novice researcher to appreciate what this process feels like. As Gide (1926) wrote in *The Counterfeiters* 'One doesn't discover new lands without consenting to lose sight of the shore for a very long time'. The same goes for the qualitative researcher. You need to be prepared to explore your data, be uncertain with your data, approach it in new ways, and challenge it with new concepts and ideas if you are really going to get to grips with data complication. It's worth swimming with the sharks if, as a result, you come up with a new contribution to your subject area.

Specific approaches to qualitative analysis

One of the exciting (or frustrating) aspects of qualitative research is that there are so many different perspectives on how things should be done. Some researchers believe that a particular methodological approach lends itself to only one particular analytical approach and any other approach would corrupt and devalue the data and subsequent findings. This school of thought sees purity of method/analysis as being one way of ensuring the quality, consistency and internal coherence of the study. Others, however, propose that there are many different methods and approaches to data analysis that could be employed with the decision being made once the researcher has 'played' with their data in different analytical ways. Coffey and Atkinson (1996: 3) propose:

> *... there are multiple practices, methods, and possibilities of analysis that qualitative researchers may employ. What links all the approaches is a central concern with transforming and interpreting qualitative data — in a rigorous and scholarly way — in order to capture the complexities of the social world we seek to understand.*

A potentially heretical comment to make is that whilst different analytical approaches claim to be doing very different jobs, the processes are often very similar (ie. reduction, display and complication). If you have chosen to undertake your analysis within a particular analytical framework, then you will need to look beyond this chapter for more detailed information to support your specific analytical approach. Constant comparative method, narrative analysis, discourse analysis and protocol analysis are all examples of (fairly) specific analytical frameworks that are used with reasonable regularity. Yet even within these approaches there is a great deal of dispute and you will often read strongly divergent expert opinion about the way to undertake analysis using a particular framework. However, for most mortals, thematic analysis (if undertaken well) is more than 'good-enough.' In addition, good thematic analysis is often more honest and more satisfactory than a badly executed attempt at a more complex analytical approach. To a certain extent, the nature of your data guides you towards some particular approaches and away from others.

For example, if you had collected stories (or narratives) from women about their experiences of attending a midwifery-led unit then you would probably be drawn to one of the narrative analysis approaches (eg. Riessman 1993; Frank 2000).

Alternatively, if your study aimed to generate hypotheses and theories you would probably be using grounded theory (Glaser and Strauss, 1967): as such, your analytical strategy would be constant comparative method. Pidgeon (1996: 78) states that within constant comparison the 'principal analytical task is one of continually sifting and comparing elements throughout the lifetime of a research project... to promote conceptual and theoretical development'.

Potter (1996: 129) states that, 'discourse analysis focuses on talk and texts as social practices and on the resources that are drawn upon to enable those practices.' Therefore, you might choose discourse analysis as the means of illuminating how talk between members of the multidisciplinary team can marginalise refugee women.

If your study aimed to determine the types of processes used by expert and student midwives in relation to client advocacy then you might choose to utilise a form of protocol (think-aloud) analysis (Green and Gillhooly, 1996).

There are now increasing numbers of papers that demonstrate how the same data can be analysed in different ways. These papers are part confessional, in as much as they demonstrate an experienced researcher returning to data they analysed in a less sophisticated manner earlier in their research careers. They do make interesting reading and help to illuminate different levels of interpretation and also demonstrate how the skills of the researcher influence the level of meaning that can be generated from the same materials (eg. Boeije, 2002; Savage, 2000). In some ways these papers illustrate and reflect the choices that all researchers make in terms of analytical approaches. Denzin and Lincoln (1996: 2–3) draw on Lévi-Strauss' (1966) notion of bricoleur as a 'Jack of all trades' when they describe the qualitative researcher-as-bricoleur who:

> *... uses the tools of his or her methodological trade, deploying whatever*
> *strategies, methods, or empirical materials as are at hand.... if new tools*
> *have to be invented, or pieced together, then the researcher will do this.*
> *... The product of the bricoleur's labor is a bricolage, a complex, dense,*
> *reflexive, collagelike creation that represents the researcher's images,*
> *understandings, and interpretations of the world or the phenomenon under*
> *analysis.*

Even if you have chosen a specific approach there is often a lack of consensus as to the definition, techniques and modes of analysis within that approach. This reflects that qualitative analysis is, to a large extent, still emerging with different researchers using their own terms and frameworks.

Computers, software packages and other 'techy' bits

> *Computers make good friends. No matter how stupid, dull or dumb we may*
> *feel, we can still feel smarter than our computer. Computers can do many*
> *things, but they cannot think — and we can. Unfortunately, that also means*
> *the thinking is up to us.*

Dey, 1995: 55

However sophisticated the qualitative analysis software package you install on your computer, it won't analyse your data. The packages are good at some of the mechanical aspects of data management but they don't allow you to feed in your data, go for a cup of tea and come back fifteen minutes later with the analysis complete. As described earlier, analysis is complex, iterative, and creative. These aspects of the intellectual process all come from the brain of the researcher (Webb, 1999). Lee and Esterhuizen (2000) talk of the shift between the perception in the 1980s of the computer as an 'alien device with roots firmly based in the quantitative paradigm' (p. 231) to becoming 'more socially accepted among qualitative researchers' (p. 232). While manual, as opposed to computer assisted, data analysis is perfectly feasible for even quite large studies, such packages are increasingly seen as a potentially powerful ally in helping manage data. The arguments that software packages and computers reduce the degree to which you can engage with and get close to your data are now less to do with the awkwardness of the early programmes, but more to do with whether or not the researcher feels comfortable with using software assistance or prefers to work manually with pen and paper. Lee and Esterhuizen (2000: 234) propose that, if used appropriately, computers can reduce the risk of researchers becoming overwhelmed by their data and can help them find an effective way of navigating and getting close to their data. However, tensions still exist and there is active debate about the methodological dangers of using computers in qualitative research (Kelle, 1997).

Most qualitative software packages can assist the researcher to undertake a number of different tasks and these, Froggatt (2001b) states, include:

* ❖ 'naming and labelling sections of the data;
* ❖ attachment of codes to segments of data;
* ❖ retrieval of all data in any code;
* ❖ attachment of analytical memos to specific codes or text;
* ❖ text searches for words, phrases or segments of text;
* ❖ Boolean searches (eg. AND/OR/NOT);
* ❖ sorting and organizing data segments;
* ❖ identifying relationships between codes;
* ❖ preparing diagrams;
* ❖ extracting quotes for illustrative purposes.'

Before leaping straight into the decision that you are going to use a software package, it is vital that you really understand the process by which you intend to analyse your data. If you do not do this you will end up having to climb two steep learning curves at the same time: curve 1, the complex process of data analysis and curve 2, the software package and its complexities. This may not be a recipe for disaster but it's certainly a recipe for additional stress and you may end up 'lost in hyperspace' (Dey, 1995: 78). For many beginning novice researchers the most appropriate option is to cut your teeth on manual analysis of data within your first project and then move on to learning and using a software package (Webb, 1999).

With any software package, the decision is whether or not it will help or hinder the analysis of your data (Morison and Moir, 1998). If it will genuinely liberate you from the mechanical aspects of data handling and free up more time to spend on the creative, intellectual analytical processes, the decision is likely to be to use the software. Most software manufacturers have demonstration versions of their software and it is worth trialing these or gaining some hands on experience of different packages before deciding which package is for you or a particular research study. The CAQDAS Networking Project (http://www.soc.surrey.ac.uk/caqdas/) offers good internet resources, and a range of other support including training courses. In summary, Richards and Richards (1994: 170) state:

> *The computer can assist, by holding a myriad of threads, exploring the sticky links to other categories, by allowing the exploration of many patterns and the building of one web on another, and of testing the strength of the resultant fabric. But the task of theory discovery remains for the human researchers; the questions are theirs, the combinations of categories specified by them. They see the links and draw the threads together, often by creative leaps or imaginative analogies or sheer field research luck, factors that have little to do with the carefully constructed index.*

Voice recognition software is unlikely to have actual analytical implications although it could potentially (when the software is further developed) replace the need for human transcription. Digital audio recording opens up many possibilities and advantages (Stockdale, 2002). Lee and Esterhuizen (2000: 238) propose that digitised audio and video (which allows you to listen to coded data rather than just read it) could have fairly major implications for the way in which data are analysed as it has 'considerable potential for speeding up at least some kinds of analysis'. In terms of computer assistance the future is likely to be exciting and contentious.

Conclusion

Having read all the way through this chapter (or having saved time by skipping straight to the conclusion!) you may be wondering why anyone would consciously choose to undertake qualitative data analysis. However, ask yourself the following questions. Have you got the heart and stamina of an explorer? Have you got untapped reserves of dogged determination? Do you relish the prospect of swimming in 'shark-infested custard'? If the answer to any of the previous questions is 'yes', then you and qualitative data analysis are more than likely to get on fine together.

Qualitative data analysis is not the soft option for people who would rather avoid statistics 'because they're difficult'. Qualitative data analysis is also difficult, albeit differently difficult. Using a qualitative approach to analysing your data opens up new vistas and new ways of thinking about things that you may take for granted. It not only provides a way of analysing your research data, it will ultimately help you to start to think about your practice, your own beliefs and assumptions in new ways.

Qualitative data analysis does require you to be a determined explorer. Occasionally you will feel as if you are out of your depth and about to drown in your own data. But, as your findings start to emerge during the processes of analysis, you will develop a liking for data exploration and you'll find yourself saying, quietly at first, 'Bring on more sharks – I can deal with them. And how about a second helping of custard!'

References

Attride-Stirling J (2001) Thematic networks: an analytic tool for qualitative research. *Qualitative Res* **1**(3): 385–405

Aubusson P (2002) Using metaphor to make sense and build theory in qualitative analysis. *The Qualitative Report* **7**(4). Online at: http://www.nova.edu/sss/QR/QR7-4/aubussion.html

Boeije H (2002) A purposeful approach to the constant comparative method in the analysis of qualitative interviews. *Qual Quantity* **36**: 391–409

Cheek J (1999) Influencing practice or simply esoteric? Researching health care using post-modern approaches. *Qualitative Health Res* **9**: 383–92

Clarke JB (1999) Hermeneutic analysis: a qualitative decision trail. *Int J Nurs Stud* **36**: 363–69

Coffey A, Atkinson P (1996) Making Sense of Qualitative Data. Complementary Research Strategies. Sage Publications, Thousand Oaks

Denzin NK, Lincoln YS (1996) Introduction: Entering the field of qualitative research. In: Denzin NK, Lincoln YS, eds. *Handbook of Qualitative Research*. Sage Publications, Thousand Oaks: 1–17

Dey I (1993) *Qualitative Data Analysis. A user friendly guide for social scientists*. Routledge, London

Dey I (1995) Reducing fragmentation in qualitative research. In: Kelle U, ed. *Computer–Aided Qualitative Data Analysis*. Theory, Methods and Practice. Sage, London

Frank AW (2000) The standpoint of storyteller. *Qualitative Health Res* **10**(3): 354–65

Froggatt KA (2001a) The analysis of qualitative data: processes and pitfalls. *Palliative Med* **15**: 433–38

Froggatt KA (2001b) Using computers in the analysis of qualitative data. *Palliative Med* **15**: 517–20

Gide A (1926) The Counterfeiters.

Glaser B, Strauss A (1967) *The Discovery of Grounded Theory*. Aldine, Chicago

Green C, Gilhooly K (1996) Protocol analysis: practical implementation. In: Richardson JTE, ed. *Handbook of Qualitative Research Methods for Psychology and the Social Sciences*. BPS Books, Leicester: 55–74

Huberman AM, Miles MB (1994) Data Management and Analysis Methods. In: Denzin NK, Lincoln YS, eds. *Handbook of Qualitative Research*. Sage Publications, Thousand Oaks: 428–44

Kelle U (1997) Theory building in qualitative research and computer programs for the management of textual data. *Sociological Research Online* **2**(2). http://www.socresonline. org.uk/socresonline/2/2/1.html

Lapadat JC (2000) Problematizing transcription: purpose, paradigm and quality. *Int J Soc Res Methodology* **3**(3): 203–19

Lee RM, Esterhuizen L (2000) Computer software and qualitative analysis: trends, issues and resources. *Int J Soc Soc Res Methodology* **3**(3): 231–43

Lévi-Strauss C (1966) *The Savage Mind*. 2nd edn. University of Chicago Press, Chicago

Mason J (1996) *Qualitative Researching*. Sage Publications, London

Meadows LM, Morse JM (2001) Constructing evidence within the qualitative project. In: Morse JM, Swanson JM, Kuzel AJ, eds. *The Nature of Qualitative Evidence*. Sage Publications, Thousand Oaks

Miles MB, Huberman AM (1994) *Qualitative Data Analysis*. 2nd edn. Sage Publications, Thousand Oaks

Morison M, Moir J (1998) The role of computer software in the analysis of qualitative data: efficient clerk, research assistant or Trojan horse? *J Adv Nurs* **28**(1): 106–16

Pidgeon N (1996) Grounded theory: theoretical background. In: Richardson JTE, ed. *Handbook of Qualitative Research Methods for Psychology and the Social Sciences*. BPS Books, Leicester: 75–85

Potter J (1996) Discourse analysis and constructionist approaches: theoretical background. In: Richardson JTE, ed. *Handbook of Qualitative Research Methods for Psychology and the Social Sciences*. BPS Books, Leicester: 125–40

Riessman CK (1993) *Narrative Analysis*. Sage, Newbury Park, CA

Riessman CK (2002) Illness Narratives: Positioned Identities. Invited annual lecture. Health Communication Research Centre, Cardiff University, Wales, UK. May. Online at: http://www.cf.ac.uk/encap/hcrc/comet/prog/narratives.pdf

Richards L, Richards T (1994) From filing cabinet to computer. In: Bryman A, Burgess RB, eds. *Analyzing Qualitative Data*. Routledge, London

Savage J (2000) One voice, different tunes; issues raised by dual analysis of a segment of qualitative data. *J Adv Nurs* **31**(6): 1439–1500

Seale C (1999) *The Quality of Qualitative Research*. Sage Publications, London

Silverman D (1993) *Interpreting Qualitative Data. Methods for Analysing Talk, Text and Interaction*. Sage Publications, London

Stockdale A (2002) Tools for digital audio recording in qualitative research. Social Research Update. 38. Online at: http://www.soc.surrey.ac.uk/sru/SRU38.html

Webb C (1999) Analysing qualitative data: computerized and other approaches. *J Adv Nurs* **29**(2): 323–30

Chapter 7

Embedding a qualitative approach within a quantitative framework: an example in a sensitive setting

Claire Snowdon, Diana Elbourne and Jo Garcia

> *Words are but images of matter, to fall in love*
> *with them is to fall in love with a picture*
> Frances Bacon, 1561–1626

Introduction

Quantitative and qualitative research methods have been regarded historically as methodological opposites. The metaphor of the battleground has commonly been used to characterise the debate on the legitimacy of the methods and validity of the data produced, with opponents being seen as 'paradigm warriors' (Tashakkori and Teddle, 1998; Oakley, 2000). While quantitative researchers are often said to charge qualitative research with being unscientific and subjective (Pope and Mays, 1995ii), Oakley (1998) has argued that 'notions of experimentation, random allocation and quantitative methods are like a red rag to a bull for many social scientists'. Although there is still some suspicion between the camps, there is a growing movement towards drawing upon the two approaches to produce research that is richer, more sensitive and adds to knowledge in a more effective way than with one method alone (Pope and Mays, 1995i; Kelle, 2001). An area in which cooperative research is flourishing is the randomised controlled trial (RCT), 'the epitome of the quantitative method' (Pope and Mays, 1995i). In the past thirty years, there has been a move towards integrating quantitative and qualitative approaches to understand better the conditions created by the use of RCTs. As a result, RCTs are now providing the context for a progressive and developing field of research.

Qualitative research and the randomised controlled trial

Randomised controlled trials can provide the most reliable and unbiased form of scientific evidence for assessing the relative effectiveness of different treatments. Theoretical discussions and reflections of ethicists, clinicians and trialists indicate that the experimental methods used in RCTs result in a major shift in the basis of care: individualised care is replaced by random allocation of treatment, participants may receive placebo, they may be required to undergo additional tests or monitoring. Such a shift may not be particularly significant in trials in relatively benign settings, such as interventions in minor ailments and information-giving processes. Many trials, however, are involved in pushing forward the boundaries of care in life-threatening or life-changing situations, such as cancer treatment, obstetrics and intensive care. In such settings, where experimentation and life events are brought together, even the smallest change in practice may affect outcomes or alter fundamentally the experiences of those involved. RCTs are essentially quantitative studies with the potential to change people's lives.

Given the primacy of the quantitative methods involved, RCTs could be considered diametrically opposed to qualitative methods of interview and detailed analysis. Nevertheless, scientists who carry out RCTs are increasingly working with qualitatively-orientated colleagues and an entire field of research has arisen to understand better the impact of research on participants and to improve the quality of trials. Despite this movement, it is commonly stated in research papers that little attention has been paid to the views of those involved in trials. There is, in fact, a substantial literature which has, over time, provided a growing understanding of many facets of trial participation, and which has increased in both sophistication and methodological rigour. Trialists and other researchers have placed a range of almost eclectic information derived from a wide variety of sources and methods into the public domain. There are, for instance, simple elements of trial data, such as correlations between demographics and acceptance or refusal rates (van Bergen *et al*, 1995), observations of trialists drawn from their experiences with patients (Dobkin, 1990; Walterspiel, 1990) and with colleagues (Klein *et al*, 1995), and many questionnaire-based and, more recently, interview-based studies in the field. The literature has been reviewed from various perspectives — Edwards *et al*, 1998 (ethics of trials); Ross *et al*, 1999, and Cox, 2003 (barriers to participation); Sugarman *et al*, 1999 (informed consent); Ellis, 2000 (attitudes to participation) — and is drawn upon below.

Typically, the earlier research on RCTs was not qualitative, or used qualitative data in a rather limited way. There were a number of studies that tried to gain an understanding of broad issues, such as general views of research and why people did or did not participate in RCTs (eg. Hassar and Weintraub, 1976; Barofsky and Sugarbaker, 1979; Henzlova *et al*, 1994). Rather than considering the particular conditions created by individual trials, studies often recruited samples of participants or non-participants (Penman *et al*, 1984) and professionals (Taylor *et al*, 1994) from several different trials, exploring elements of participation as if the trials constituted a single, coherent entity. Studies involving members of the public (Cassileth *et al*, 1982; Kemp *et al*, 1984) or patients with no experience of trial participation (Llewellyn-Thomas *et al*, 1991; Mettlin *et al*, 1985; Saurbrey *et al*, 1984) produced data on attitudes to trials that were essentially hypothetical.

Some researchers did explore the conditions of individual trials (Henzlova *et al*, 1984; Howard *et al*, 1981). An important theme in both early and more recent research is assessment of patient-centred obstacles to recruitment (Smith and Arnesen, 1988; Tait *et al*, 1998; Mohanna and Tunna, 1999; Dorantes *et al*, 2000; Jenkins and Fallowfield, 2000; Salomons *et al*, 2002) to try to explain why the trials involved had failed and/or to improve future recruitment rates. Some trialists reported on the impact of the views or behaviour of physicians on the progress of their trials (Tognoni *et al*, 1991; Klein *et al*, 1995). Klein *et al* (1995), for example, found that obstetricians involved in a trial of episiotomy frequently overrode random allocation where it conflicted with their own judgement of the management of labour. Some trialists reported elements of their trial data that shed some light on patients' reactions to the constraints of the research setting. Abramsky and Rodeck (1990) reported drop-out rates due to patient dissatisfaction on allocation in a trial comparing chorion villus sampling (CVS) to amniocentesis, and Williams *et al* (1980) reported poor compliance in a trial on ambulation in labour. It became clear that if a trial is not acceptable to professionals or does not meet patients' needs, it may be doomed to fail with low levels of recruitment or high drop-out rates.

Although some of the earlier work was limited, and methods of reporting data have at times been problematic (see Edwards *et al*, 1998, for a critique), the insights gained from the early studies and the reports from trials provided the basis and impetus for a wave of qualitative studies, and over the years much ground has been covered. Qualitative researchers developed an interest in understanding more about exactly how trials influence the experiences of those involved. As the reports described above demonstrated, the factors that render a trial attractive or unattractive to patients, or to those responsible for recruitment, may not be immediately obvious to those involved in running a trial. Uncovering these factors and valuing participant experiences became an area for some of the earlier qualitative studies. Ryan (1995), for instance, used in-depth interviews to understand the difficulties for men participating in an HIV trial and found that a particular problem for participants was having to visit the clinic for the trial. These visits made participants' HIV status explicit to other attenders, and implied sexual orientation. Some asymptomatic participants were disconcerted by encounters with other attenders in a more advanced stage of the disease, thus making trial participation difficult, or even unacceptable.

Informed consent is central to the ethical management of RCTs and the study of the quality and meaning of consent has grown over the years. Although there are many questionnaire-based studies (eg. van Stuijvenberg *et al*, 1998; Tait *et al*, 1998; Ferguson, 2002; Burgess *et al*, 2003), there has been a rise in the number of interview-based studies that have explored this area (eg. Gray, 1975; Appelbaum *et al*, 1987; Snowdon *et al*, 1997, 1999; Featherstone and Donovan, 1998; Cox, 1999, 2000; Mason *et al*, 2000; Featherstone and Donovan, 2002; Glogowska *et al*, 2001; Mills *et al*, 2003). Whilst qualitative data can be used to add breadth to quantitative data, in these circumstances they have proved to be invaluable in allowing a deeper, more meaningful understanding of circumstances that could not have been tapped by quantitative methods alone. This is demonstrated by Featherstone and Donovan (2002) who carried out in-depth, semi-structured interviews with men who had been offered participation in a urology trial. They found important misconceptions about the trial through their analysis and argued that a structured questionnaire would have been an inappropriate and potentially misleading tool, given the subtlety of the data generated. '[I]t is likely that the majority of these participants would have been shown to be aware that they were taking part in a trial and to have understood some or most of the basic aspects of the design.'

Whilst researchers have frequently commented retrospectively on one trial to improve practice in subsequent trials, more recently qualitative research has been carried out to guide and effect practical changes in an existing trial. Donovan *et al* (2002) carried out a radical qualitative study using action-research methods in which men were randomly assigned to different recruitment procedures for a prostate-treatment trial. The results of the findings from in-depth interviews, analysis of the audio-taped recruitment appointments, and follow-up interviews brought about crucial practical changes in the management of the trial. They found that there were difficulties for the professionals involved in recruitment in discussing the basis for the trial (uncertainty over treatment or 'equipoise') and in presenting treatments without bias or terminology that would be subsequently misinterpreted by participants. This information was used to modify the trial procedures. Not only did the insights from the qualitative study bring about important changes to the information processes to promote participant understanding, the trial itself also benefited from an increase in the randomisation rate from 40% to 70%. The authors argue persuasively for the value of their approach: 'qualitative research methods applied in combination with open minded clinicians and flexible or innovative trial designs may enable even the most difficult evaluative questions to be tackled and have substantial impacts even on apparently routine and uncontroversial trials'.

The use of qualitative research to aid interpretation of the results of trials also marks a significant milestone in the collaboration between trialists and qualitative researchers. Describing their research as 'a multimethod approach', Glogowska *et al* (2002) used questionnaires and interviews with parents of preschool children involved in a speech and language therapy trial, and combined these with data from the RCT. The quantitative trial results suggested that the trial had shown the intervention to be ineffective. The qualitative study demonstrated parents' perceptions of important advantages, as well as limitations, that the authors felt that they 'could only have surmised from the pragmatic trial alone'.

The growth and increase in the quality of qualitative studies in this area of experimental medicine is important. People have been participating in RCTs for over fifty years and still further research is necessary to understand better many aspects of their perspectives. This is especially the case in trials in particularly sensitive settings, such as labour and delivery, surgery, mental health care, the treatment of life-threatening illnesses or emergency settings, where potential participants or their proxies may be expected to be particularly vulnerable. It is precisely because areas such as these are so powerfully charged, both emotionally and politically, that research into attitudes to, and experiences of, participation is sorely needed but difficult to implement. The integration of two types of research in the one setting is challenging. It requires political will and dedicated co-operation between researchers from diverse professional backgrounds (Chalmers 1998).

This chapter provides an extended description of a challenging aspect of a qualitative study, that is recruitment and interviews with bereaved parents involved in an RCT in the setting of neonatal intensive care. Trials in this highly stressful setting can be particularly difficult (Manning 2000) and where babies go on to die parents are often especially vulnerable. The chapter focuses on the development of our research processes, some illustrative findings (researching research) and reflections upon parental involvement in our own research (researching research that researches research), showing insights from our qualitative approach.

The ECMO qualitative studies — a developmental approach

The first in a series of qualitative studies assessed trial participation from the perspectives of parents of babies involved in the UK Collaborative Trial of Extra Corporeal Membrane Oxygenation (ECMO) (Snowdon *et al*, 1997). The trial involved critically ill new-born babies, and compared two methods of life-support: 'conventional' management (involving ventilatory support) versus oxygenation of the blood via an external circuit (UK Collaborative ECMO Trial Group, 1996). Subsequent studies were carried out with an additional group of ECMO trial parents (Snowdon *et al*, 1998,

1999), with health professionals and parents linked to four trials (see below), and with health professionals and parents of babies undergoing hypothermia and ECMO in a pre-trial study (Snowdon *et al*, unpublished). At each stage of the process there were critical insights which both informed the findings and shaped subsequent research topics. These various studies therefore represent an intellectual and a methodological progression.

The early studies involved only parents of surviving babies. At the time the published research on the views of participants in trials was more limited and there was little to guide research in such a sensitive area. Whilst research on bereavement was available, it was important to consider that trial participation was an added and potentially complicating dimension. It was very difficult to predict the likely impact of some of the discussions required for the interviews. It was decided that although the views of bereaved parents were potentially valuable, it was inappropriate to include these parents when the field was so limited and when the research team was exploring essentially new research territory.

The most instructive finding from the first study was the demonstration of the difficulties that parents of surviving babies had in describing aspects of the trial. It was clear that even where parents were familiar with RCT terminology, they were often uncertain about the nature of randomisation and the rationale behind its use. Whilst the stressful and emotional circumstances of the discussion of the trial are likely to have hindered the transmission and receipt of complicated information, it was interesting to find that there were some consistent misconceptions about the trial that recurred in different interviews around the country. It seemed likely that some particular accounts may have had their roots in formal and informal conversations with staff involved in the trial. Some were natural and common sense responses to crucial gaps in knowledge. For instance, some parents (understandably) did not have an appreciation of medical uncertainty as the basis for the trial. They then sought other means to explain the use of randomisation, such as a means of circumventing a difficult decision for doctors to choose which treatment a baby should have, or as a means of deciding between babies competing for scarce ECMO beds. Where the evaluative nature of a trial was not clear, some parents believed their sick baby was deprived of a known life-saving therapy. Allocation to conventional management was taken by some parents to mean that their baby had been 'rejected'. Views such as these have implications both for the management of trials and for the well-being of participants and their proxies.

The subsequent ECMO qualitative studies also gave useful insights, allowing the team to develop further research questions and methodological approaches. They showed that parents largely valued their involvement in a trial, in particular, being informed about the trial once the results were available (Snowdon *et al*, 1998), and that it was possible to explore with parents their attitudes to methodological issues, namely an alternative approach to consent for trials (Snowdon *et al*, 1999). The studies provide information which may be used by trialists to reflect on management issues for their research.

The results of the ECMO Trial studies have been widely disseminated, both in publications and presentations. A very frequent response from audiences, and in print (Braunholz, 1999; Manning, 2000), has been to comment that results may have been different had bereaved parents been included in the study. As researchers we were frequently called upon to defend the decision to include only parents of surviving babies in this earlier research. Although this decision was described as being based on 'perfectly understandable ethical reasons' (Braunholtz, 1999), it was clear that there was a need to understand the impact of trial participation on those with a very difficult outcome, and to assess their experiences both at the time and with hindsight. It was decided that the team had gained sufficient experience and understanding of the field to incorporate an assessment of the views of bereaved parents into a subsequent study.

The study of views of participants in perinatal trials

For this study the wider aim was to examine issues associated with trial participation from the perspectives of doctors, midwives, neonatal nurses, parents of babies that survived (including parents who had declined trial participation) and parents of babies that died. The setting was two neonatal RCTs, the INNOVO Trial (Field *et al*, (submitted); www.innovo-trial.org.uk) and the CANDA Trial (Ainsworth *et al*, 2000), both of which involved critically ill babies with a high risk of mortality; and two antenatal trials, the TEAMS Trial (Brocklehurst *et al*, 1999) and ORACLE (Kenyon *et al*, 2001a; Kenyon *et al*, 2001b). Although the original aim was to carry out interviews with bereaved parents who had been offered any of the four trials, difficulties arose in some centres where access to bereaved parents was not permitted, especially in the antenatal trials. The decision was eventually made to approach only parents of survivors in the two antenatal trials and so the following information is based on parents involved in one or both of the two neonatal trials.

A sensitive setting

The interviews for this research can be considered to be sensitive in a number of ways. Firstly, they involve potentially vulnerable people and every effort must be made to offer them respect and protection, even if this means accepting a degree of compromise in the data.

Secondly, the interviews are sensitive because of the subject under exploration. Not only is information about trial participation embedded within the story of the birth and death of their baby, the interviews also needed careful management because they involved exploration of the potential of the RCT for changing the parental experience. This could be in relatively small ways, such as satisfaction with information giving, or it could be in explosive and life-changing ways, such as the feeling that doctors were denying a dying baby a potentially useful treatment.

Thirdly, we had to be aware that the study itself had the potential to change the parental experience. Our earlier research had shown that parents could often use the terminology associated with a trial and appear to have a good appreciation of trial methods, but on further exploration could hold co-existing views which were at odds with the experimental rationale, such as feeling that their doctor influenced randomisation in some way to ensure access to an experimental treatment for their baby. As interviewers we had to be careful to explore parental views without interrupting their coping mechanisms, and without revealing information which might be difficult to integrate into their accounts of events, such as the random nature of the allocation. If parents felt reassured that a doctor had selected the best treatment it would be inappropriate to introduce during an interview the role that chance had played in events.

The course of the study

This degree of sensitivity affected the course of the study in significant ways. Although there had been concern expressed in the field that research that did not represent bereaved parents was fundamentally flawed, it proved to be extremely difficult to secure co-operation with other professionals and to recruit this element of the sample. From the start of the study there was a tension between support for the need to assess the impact of RCTs on bereaved parents, and concern that in researching their views, the qualitative study could undermine their wellbeing. The means by which potential participants were approached and invited to join the study was necessarily modified during the study in response to the concerns of research ethics committees (RECs) and clinicians, and to the practicalities of gaining access to the parents. REC approval was a lengthy process, often involving several RECs with different responses, and negotiations with representatives of hospital bodies (such as the Caldecott Guardians) and with the staff involved also proved to be highly problematic at times. Some clinicians were very supportive and clearly wished to see the data in the public domain. They offered much support and advice. Others, however, had misgivings. One clinician advised colleagues in a meeting not to join unless they were prepared to find themselves under media scrutiny once results were available. In some cases a departmental decision was made to permit the study in their centre, but individuals were uncomfortable and withheld access to bereaved parents once REC approval had been given and the study was underway. It seemed that we were attempting to provide the research data that everyone agreed was necessary but few felt able to support in practice. Whilst it was clear to all involved that the qualitative research must not be to the detriment of the parents involved, ultimately these concerns limited the potential for the study to answer the research questions posed.

Where an approach to bereaved parents was agreed, this was negotiated by the local hospital consultant who would raise the possibility of contact with the research team either at a bereavement visit, by letter or by telephone, according to local preferences. This required a degree of methodological flexibility and necessitated a number of modifications to multi-centre and local REC approval. If parents gave permission for this contact, they were sent a letter regarding the qualitative study.

In a gradual and slow process, twenty-one letters were sent to bereaved parents (sixteen INNOVO and five CANDA). No reminder letters were sent, at the request of the RECs. Eleven interviews were carried out with eighteen parents of thirteen babies who had died (seven INNOVO and four CANDA). The interviews were carried out by CS (8), MM (2) and DE (1). All interviews took place in the parental home, were tape recorded and fully transcribed, with the exception of one tape which was corrupted. Given the small numbers it is inappropriate to use these data to attempt to generalise about what parents might think. Instead, the parental experiences can be used to encourage reflection on research processes. Four cases are presented here in detail, two of which give some insights into the experiences of those with difficult outcomes in a quantitative study, and two which helped us to reflect on our own management of qualitative research.

Reflections on participating in the quantitative study (the INNOVO Trial)

In the ECMO qualitative study interviews, parents described their reactions to an extremely distressing situation. Their babies were critically ill and a doctor described an intervention that could potentially make a difference, but which was potentially associated with some as yet unevaluated risks. The trial compared the intervention to the control of continuing with standard care; allocation to receive standard care was almost invariably met with emotions ranging from disappointment to extreme distress. It was common for the parents of babies allocated to ECMO who survived to comment that it would have been very difficult to cope had the baby been allocated to the standard care and had not survived. This particular issue was also frequently raised by professionals when discussing the trials, but there was no research evidence to aid understanding of the possible perspectives of bereaved parents in this position.

The inclusion of bereaved parents from the INNOVO trial offered an opportunity to start exploring the issue of the impact of trial participation on those with a difficult outcome. This trial involved a relatively simple intervention, adding a gas (nitric oxide) to those already received via a ventilator. In contrast, in the ECMO trial, the intervention involved transfer to another hospital and a high-technology, highly invasive life support system. In the early stages of the study we were repeatedly advised that although both trials involved critically ill babies and a comparison with standard care, the interventions were so different that the circumstances were not comparable. In fact, the experiences of the trial reported by parents were remarkably similar. The crucial factor was the potential of an intervention, whatever that might be, to save a baby's life. Parents in the INNOVO Trial, just like those in the ECMO Trial, reported feelings of elation and relief at allocation to receive the experimental arm (nitric oxide) and disappointment, anger and regret on allocation to the control arm of the trial. Parents of survivors similarly expressed their sympathy with bereaved parents.

Eight of the interviews involved bereaved parents of babies enrolled in the INNOVO Trial (the CANDA Trial involved a comparison of two very similar treatments and is not considered in this section). Four of the babies were allocated to receive nitric oxide, three were allocated to standard care (ie. no nitric oxide), and in one case the parents did not recall the allocation. Those who received the treatment were very positive about the trial and felt that they could be confident that everything had been tried in order to save their baby. They felt both that the doctors had exhausted all options, and that as parents they too had exercised their responsibilities and ensured that all avenues had been explored. It is possible that a larger sample might uncover parents who worried that their decision to permit the use of an experimental intervention had a role in their baby's death but this was not the case here. The experimental nature of the drug was almost irrelevant, with one mother stating: 'it didn't really matter that it was a trial, it was a fact that anything would help'. Those who did not receive nitric oxide were however in quite a different situation.

Dawn and Peter[1]

Dawn gave birth to twins six weeks early. They were both in a poor condition and had contracted an infection (no further details given in the interview). One baby, Amy, was

---

1.   All names are pseudonyms.

enrolled in the INNOVO Trial and was allocated to the control group. Both babies were christened in hospital and Amy died after six days. During the interview Dawn and Peter took turns holding their surviving baby, Catherine (who had not been eligible for enrolment in the trial) who is affected by a number of health problems. Sometimes she slept and sometimes they stroked or fed her. They both displayed a lot of affection which may have helped them as they recalled painful times. It may also have helped to avoid eye contact with the interviewer and gave everyone a helpful channel for positive comments.

Their description of the events surrounding their consent to join the INNOVO Trial was somewhat disjointed. They described how the consultant who offered the trial to them had characterized the situation. Dawn repeatedly focused on what was for her the most important element of what she said the consultant had told them, 'It's her last chance. If she doesn't get it she'll probably die anyway, ... but if she gets this she's getting a last chance.' Peter gave a description of the consultant's explanation of why the use of nitric oxide was randomised as, 'some doctors think it does work, some think it's nothing to do with that, the babies just pick up'. It seemed as if the drug was being randomized because doctors could not agree whether it was useful or not. Whilst this is not at all far from the truth, there was a subtle implication that this was largely a way to manage uncertainty. They did not present the trial as in any way evaluative or as a form of limiting exposure to an untested drug and this was a crucial element in their description of their experiences. Dawn felt that, 'everyone should get the chance at it.'

The news that Amy had been allocated to standard care was devastating. With the experimental element of the intervention out of the equation, and with nitric oxide being seen as the last available route, the parents felt that they were left 'just sitting there watching her die'. They felt that the process was particularly cruel, 'a totally horrible thing to do'. The key element in their experience was a sense of having a potential solution dangled in front of them, a solution which they felt their doctor was powerless to access. They felt that he too was upset at the allocation. Peter made it clear that he did not hold their consultant responsible, saying 'we never blamed [him]. It's somewhere else along the line isn't it where all that comes from. It's not the doctors at the hospitals.'

There was a definite sense that an important option had not been explored. Dawn said, 'they'd done everything they could but that random thingy.' At times this interview felt quite desolate and the loss of their baby was completely at the forefront of their lives. Poloroid photographs of the twin girls in their incubators had been substantially enlarged and were on display, an intensely sad reminder of the circumstances of their loss. The most poignant comment in the interview came from Dawn, in making a point that she returned to several times. 'That's what goes on in my head, you know, if she would have got it, maybe she might be still here.'

Erica and Howard

During pregnancy Erica and Howard were told that their baby was affected by hydrops. At thirty-four weeks Erica was hospitalised and they were made aware that the prognosis may be poor. After several days Erica went into spontaneous labour, and underwent an emergency Caesarean section with a general anaesthetic. Howard was given a brief glimpse of the baby, Jenny, as she was taken straight to neonatal intensive care. Although she was very swollen, he said that he felt that she was 'beautiful'. He spent time with her and came to see that she was 'very damaged' and did not really feel that there was much that could be done. He described her chances as 'twenty to thirty per cent' and very much felt that the deciding factor would be whether or not Jenny decided to fight for her survival, arguing that 'it was just a case of monitoring her, it was all in Jenny's court really, there was not much that they could have done really apart from drain and monitor, and then if Jenny wanted to make a go of it they could have done more.' There was however still a sense at this stage that she may survive, as they were told that the first twenty-four hours would be crucial for her.

In the meantime, Erica had developed a bowel infection. She had not seen the baby and although she had had some feedback she found it difficult to remember and could not appreciate what was happening to Jenny. Howard left the hospital and at 5.00 am Erica was woken by a doctor to discuss the possibility of enrolling Jenny in the INNOVO Trial. Jenny was critically ill and declining rapidly. A call was made to bring Howard back to the hospital, but there was no time to wait for him to arrive. Erica had to listen to the information in her bed and decide about the trial on her own. She was asked to give her decision in five minutes. She said 'I was drugged up because I was on morphine, I was sort of out of it, I didn't know what was going on.' She describes the conversation and her view of the trial as follows:

> *He came to me and said 'baby isn't well so we can do this trial' he said 'but there is only sixty in the country' or something 'and it's like picking you out of a hat', and I turned round and said 'What about her chances?' and he said to me, 'There isn't really much hope.' He said, 'She's deteriorating fast but it's up to you what you want to do' and I said, 'Go for it!'*

Erica's account of the basis of the trial includes the availability of a treatment which may or may not benefit their daughter, and that it might not be accessible. She saw the trial as involving a treatment which might help. Her focus in the discussion about the trial was solely on the potential of nitric oxide to help their situation.

> *As soon as he said that, the main thing that was stuck in my mind was anything that would help her then yeah go for it, it gave her a better chance. ... [E]ven though it was her last chance there was still hope.*

Once she gave her consent the allocation was made very quickly and Jenny was to receive nitric oxide. Howard arrived at the hospital and they went together to see her. In fact, Jenny deteriorated further and nitric oxide was not used. Howard described the timing:

> *I got there for about twenty past five and ... Erica ... [had] already given the nod about the trial about ten past and at half past five you were been wheeled in to say our goodbyes, by half past seven Jenny was dead.*

There are important technical preparations which have to be made in order to administer nitric oxide for the trial. From the details given in the interview it is not possible to say whether there was simply not enough time to make these preparations or whether Jenny was ultimately too sick to undergo any changes to her circumstances. Erica and Howard were however left with the impression that the trial involved allocation to a ventilator which had to be brought to the hospital. They felt that there had not been time to get the ventilator to them.

The parents were frustrated at the timing, feeling that they had been asked about the trial at such a late stage, despite the fact that Jenny's condition was clear from a week before she was born. Erica felt that she would have preferred to read material in advance so that a decision could have been made at an earlier stage. When Erica finally saw her daughter she realized just how ill she was. Erica accepted that she would not now receive nitric oxide and they chose to have Jenny removed from her ventilator. She found herself reflecting on their earlier fight to save her:

> *When I saw her I thought is it worth it, I mean as to what problems will she have if she does survive, there is a chance that she will be blind, they thought she had brain damage and I thought no you know what are her chances in life realistically. There's no point in prolonging her life for another couple of years, if it was going to happen I'd rather it happened there and then.*

For Howard, who described himself as 'bitter' and 'really disappointed', there was the sense that they had been lucky to gain access to the trial but that an opportunity had been missed, given what they had been told about the importance of the first twenty-four hours.

> *There was maybe one in sixty chance of getting this trial and it was all done by draws and everything else and I was thinking, you know, by the time you've decided who is going to get the trial at this late stage with Jenny she'd gone anyway. ... [I]f we'd maybe been offered any time of day before when Jenny had a chance it could go either way, great, fair do's, [but] by then she was virtually gone, ... she was damaged beyond belief, so even if you know, they would have had the chance to put her on the machine it wouldn't have done her the slightest bit of good anyway, she was gone, she was well and truly gone.*

Once home, Erica found a website on nitric oxide which made her feel that Jenny may have survived had they been offered the trial earlier. She said that she was feeling, 'What if...?'. In retrospect, Howard described the trial as potentially offering them something important but that ultimately it may have had 'a detrimental effect' in raising unrealistic expectations.

Reflections on participation in the qualitative study

These accounts demonstrate the sensitive nature of the qualitative study. Given their experiences, the topic under discussion and the concerns of some consultants who were approached for assistance with the study, it is important to reflect on participation in the qualitative study itself.

The recruitment process

The process of making the initial contact with parents was potentially problematic as there was no information as to how parents would view the offer of joining the study. After much consultation, including discussion with the parent members of the project's advisory group, it was decided that involving their consultant was crucial. Not only did this allow consultants to feel involved in the process and to offer them some reassurance that inappropriate contacts were not being pursued, it also lent a degree of credibility to the study which may have made parents feel more secure. This approach meant, however, that the initial sampling process was highly selective. Consultants were protective of the parents and not surprisingly did not give permission for approaches to families whom they expected would be particularly stressed. It was also unlikely that they would have recommended contact with those with a poor relationship with their unit. Once parents were invited to participate there was another level of selection as various parents decided whether or not to participate.

Whilst there was a concern that parents may have felt a degree of obligation to their consultant, it was reassuring that the study achieved very similar rates of agreement to participate when bereaved parents were compared to those whose babies survived. In half of the cases bereaved parents chose not to return a reply slip and were not contacted again. Although it may have resulted in a higher response rate we accepted the loss of potential data as a consequence of an appropriate ethical safeguard.

The interviews

The interviews were varied in tone, from highly charged to very comfortable. Some parents cried during the interviews and were always given the opportunity to stop for a break or to discontinue. None chose the latter. Some had a very serious tone and it was clear that we were tapping the most dreadful of experiences with which parents were still struggling. Some were more relaxed and there was a strong sense that although difficult, they felt able to talk and wanted to make their experiences known. It was obvious that the interview was a big event for which parents had often mentally prepared themselves, or had made practical preparations like arranging for their children to be looked after so that they were free to talk. Only one mother seemed very relaxed about the process. She had forgotten that the interview was booked and opened the door in her pyjamas. She was clear that she still wanted to continue and the interview went ahead while she ate breakfast. Whatever the style and tone of the interviews, parents generally seemed very committed to contributing to the research and were interested to know about our findings and the views of others with similar experiences.

As part of a monitoring process, parents who were interviewed were left a brief questionnaire which asked how they had found the interview. It was clear that the interviews could be difficult but that this was not unexpected or unacceptable. Parents seemed to welcome the opportunity to talk and one mother said that she was 'glad that I had the courage to take part'. This gives a flavour of the approach of a number of the parents, who felt that they wanted both the opportunity to talk and the chance to make their opinions known. The need to be heard was crucial for one couple, Linda and Colin, and their inclusion in the study was extremely valuable in terms of the insights it gave in to the importance of affording vulnerable groups every opportunity to opt in as well as to opt out of research into their experiences. The interview with Judith and Sean caused the researchers to worry that parents may have found the interview too stressful, exactly the concerns of some professionals.

Linda and Colin

As we were negotiating access to parents in one of the trials we were told of a consultant's decision to exclude a couple as their experience of neonatal intensive care and involvement in the trial had been extraordinarily harrowing. It was a common occurrence for such a decision to be made, but in this instance the decision was unexpectedly revoked after the consultant had a further discussion with a clinical colleague. The couple were approached, agreed to see a letter about the study and sent a signed consent form for the interview by return of post. With some knowledge of their difficult history the interviewer (CS) felt a degree of trepidation and concern that this might prove to be the most challenging interview of the study. It did, in fact, prove to be possibly the most instructive interview in the study.

Linda conceived triplets after assisted conception but her babies were delivered at twenty-four weeks after several attempts to stop labour. They were born at the lower limits of survival. The birth of the babies was complicated and confusing and the parents were left with unresolved questions about the delivery process. All three babies died over an extended period, the last baby quite unexpectedly. The parents had permitted enrollment in the CANDA trial for all three babies. They did not know to which treatment groups the babies had been allocated. The main value of this interview was that it very clearly demonstrated how much these parents wanted to be involved in both the trial and the qualitative study. They were, however, almost excluded from the qualitative study. During the interview they were asked whether they felt that it is appropriate to feed back trial results to bereaved parents, given that it might involve emotionally difficult information. Their views were very clear; Linda was almost offended at the suggestion that they should be treated differently from other parents.

> *I wouldn't like to think that because our babies died ... they feel they couldn't approach us and give us the results of the trial, whereas other folk that's been in the trial whose babies have survived, ... they would find it easier to get in contact with them and give them the result. ... They're quick enough to come to you to enrol in the trial. And just because your babies didn't survive doesn't mean to say that you're not interested. ... Why shouldn't you get the results!*

At the end of the interview they gave permission to use their information even though it was pointed out that their unique situation would probably identify them to those involved in their care. They spontaneously suggested that we could access their medical record if that would help in any way. Although this was not necessary for the qualitative study, it was a measure of their desire to co-operate and provide useful information for the research.

Claire Snowdon, Diana Elborne and Jo Garcia

Judith and Sean

This was an unexpectedly difficult interview as it was not clear until the interviewer arrived at the parents' house that Judith was approximately seven months pregnant. Their first child had died unexpectedly at full term having contracted a streptococcal infection and Judith was clearly having a stressful time, worrying that they may repeat the experience. The interview notes prepared immediately afterwards by CS capture some of the atmosphere.

> I didn't feel that any of us really relaxed and I felt uncomfortable with some of the questions that I asked. Although Judith cried during the interview, she did not want to stop. Sean had left the television playing cartoons with the sound turned down which he was watching when I arrived. It occasionally caught his attention during the interview and at those times was less engaged with the interview. There were some times when I don't think I explored things as well as I can when people are engaged with the questions or seem more comfortable. I think the fact that they did not have a healthy child left an almost unbearable feeling of sadness. When I left, for the first time ever, I regretted having done the interview and found myself questioning whether I had put this couple through something unpleasant to no benefit to themselves.

The post-interview questionnaire proved a valuable resource in resolving some of these concerns. In answer to the question, 'How did you feel afterwards?' Judith wrote 'A little upset. It brought back a lot of memories but I didn't regret talking about it'. Both Judith and Sean also ticked that there was nothing they disliked about the interview. The observed tension, and the parental willingness to tolerate emotional discussions, is a measure of their commitment to the research. Researcher concerns are an indication of the difficulties that outsiders have in tapping these most difficult experiences, even if those most affected do wish to offer their testimonies.

Although it seemed at the time that this interview had not flowed as well as others do, and it was a concern that through some degree of interviewer reticence more limited data had been collected, on analysis the interview proved particularly valuable in substantiating the views of parents in other interviews. Like many parents, Judith and Sean expressed their sense that nitric oxide represented the last option for their baby, with the comment, 'There wasn't any other treatment, it was either that or nothing really.' Judith said that although she felt some degree of caution about the fact that they would be participating in research, something 'experimental', 'we agreed to do it because we wanted to just try every, anything.' They felt very positive about the fact that nitric oxide had been tried and that had their son's infection not been so virulent, it may have saved him. This seemed to be important in both of their accounts, possibly a valuable coping mechanism. Sean, who gave a very clear description of how nitric oxide was thought to work, and who knew that there was the possibility of side effects, described how he felt positive about his involvement in the trial: 'he's been given every chance to live that he could have had then. Without the trial would we be sitting here thinking, if he'd have had it, would he be alright?'

Summary

The RCT has become a crucial tool in the move towards evidence-based medicine in the NHS and qualitative methods are increasingly being accepted in the medical community as another legitimate form of evidence (Jones, 1995). We are now seeing a significant development in which qualitative data are collected within the framework of the RCT (as opposed to explaining phenomena from an external perspective). The use of such data alongside quantitative data represents a shift to a more holistic, integrated view in which an intervention is not seen in a narrow clinical focus but in a social context. It is part of the larger trend reported here and reflects a cultural shift towards valuing the views of those who experience interventions first hand (Muir Gray, 1999).

The four cases reported here give important glimpses into the lives of those who are living with the consequences of extremely difficult experiences, and some understanding of how a trial has impacted upon their lives. They represent a group whose views have not been examined previously but who are the focus of much professional concern. Their testimonies can be used to shape future research on neonatal trials. The interview with Linda and Colin was, for instance, particularly useful in highlighting their view that it is important not to exclude bereaved parents from inclusion in an RCT because their baby has died. Clearly there is no follow-up of a baby to carry out, but bereaved parents who wish to have some continuing involvement in a trial, can be given the option of inclusion in any feed-back of results, can be sent newsletters and can be included in research in selected area such as any economic follow up (costs associated with an intervention) or any research which collects their opinions. A broader assessment of parental reactions to inclusion in such studies would be an appropriate area for a qualitative investigation.

The finding that some parents in this setting were keen to be heard is also valuable in methodological terms. It tells us that qualitative research in this area is possible and appropriate. The accounts of Dawn and Peter, and Erica and Howard, are reminders of the powerful emotions that researchers are tapping and the need for care both in trials and any associated qualitative research. There is a strong impulse to protect those who are bereaved by not raising the subject of their difficult experiences. Bereaved parents do, however, live with grief and not including them in research does not take that away. It does however take away their voice and denies them the chance to talk about experiences to an interested listener. Murray (2003) has argued that although qualitative researchers are often discouraged by 'the task of connecting with a vulnerable population and asking them to disclose information about a sensitive aspect of their lives', there can be important 'therapeutic benefits' for interviewees. We support this argument, given the positive comments made by the many parents who have taken part in our studies, but we would also wish to add that it is important not to lose sight of the potential for harm in unexpected circumstances or in certain cases. All interviews and the questions involved should be justifiable. In our interviews, some parents wanted to describe the moment of their baby's death whilst others were clearly skirting around this subject. It was important to retain the focus of the interview, participation in a trial, and to allow the parents the flexibility to revisit this experience if they so wished, but not to require them to give difficult information which was to some extent off topic. Just as researchers in trials are required to ensure that the inclusion of each participant and each intervention is necessary, it is also the case that qualitative researchers should try to ensure that each interview for a study represents an important addition to the data, either in opening new avenues of thought or in corroborating and consolidating existing findings.

Final thoughts

The material collected in the course of this part of the study is instructive, even though the sample was not collected in the coherent and consistent approach envisaged, and despite the small numbers involved. It demonstrates the importance of researchers in sensitive situations being responsive to the needs of potential participants, even if this results in certain compromises to the data. There is no doubt that the experiences described in such a difficult study as this will not be representative but we would argue that given the early stage of this element of the research field, there is an ethical imperative to explore and report such data.

At this point in the understanding of the impact of RCTs, the value of the data does not lie in their representativeness. Their importance lies in how they might be used to start to understand some of the various ways in which trial participation can affect the experiences at the centre of the research and to prompt reflection on aspects of trial management. They allow for preliminary but still important insights into the views of parents who have undergone an unfortunately not uncommon experience, but an experience that is at present under-researched. The interviews with Dawn and Peter, and Erica and Howard, not only give insights which can effect practical changes in, for instance, highlighting the possible need for support structures for parents who feel that their baby has been denied a treatment, they also provide examples of how qualitative research can highlight ethical issues which are ripe for discussion. The experiences of Erica and Howard bring to the fore two difficult issues which are highly relevant to clinicians involved in both the delivery of care and recruitment in these stressful circumstances. Firstly, when a baby is almost but not quite moribund, trials can offer a doctor access to an additional and potentially important tool which they hope will reverse their decline. At such a stage in the course of a baby's rapid deterioration clinicians have to make the difficult judgment as to whether such a slim chance of survival offsets the associated decision-making process, the limitations on parental time with their baby, raising possibly false hopes and any, as yet, inadequately evaluated consequences of allocation if they go on to be bereaved. This issue had to be faced a number of times in both the ECMO and the INNOVO trial: in the latter, three babies died before the allocated nitric oxide could be administered (Field *et al*, submitted). Secondly the interview with Erica and Howard highlights the differences between a mother's almost instinctive decision making process before she has seen her baby and connected with the full implications of fighting to save her in a damaged state, and her views on continuation of treatment once this connection has been made.

As so little is known about how bereaved parents experience involvement in trials, any exploratory data, if carefully collected and analysed, can be used to help to guide the direction of future research and to promote debate. The study is an example of how qualitative data can be used to add to knowledge and understanding through prioritising the experience of individuals, and assessing these in their larger social context.

Acknowledgements

The chapter is dedicated to the parents of CS whose own experiences are to an extent echoed here and have, over the years, shaped the research process in important ways.

References

Abramsky L, Rodeck CH (1990) Women's choices for fetal chromosome analysis. *Prenatal Diagnosis* **11**(1): 23–8

Ainsworth SB, Beresford MW, Milligan DWA *et al* (2000) Pumactant and poractant alfa for treatment of respiratory distress syndrome in neonates born at 25-29 weeks' gestation: a randomised trial. *The Lancet* **355**(9213): 1387–92

Appelbaum PS, Roth L H, Lidz CW, Benson P, Winslade W (1987) *False hopes and best data: Consent to research and the theraputic misconception.* Hastings Center Report April: 24

Barofsky I, Sugarbaker PH (1979) Determinants of patient nonparticipation in randomised clinical trials for the treatment of sarcomas. *Cancer Clinical Trials* **2**: 237–46

Braunholtz DA (1999) A note on Zelen randomization: Attitudes of parents participating in a neonatal clinical trial. *Control Clin Trials* **20**(6): 569–71

Brocklehurst P, Alfirevic Z, Chamberlain G (1999) *Protocol for the Trial of the Effects of Antenatal Multiple Courses of Steroids versus a single course.* NPEU, Oxford (see http://www.npeu.ox.ac.uk/trials/teams.html)

Burgess E, Singhal N, Amin H, McMillan DD, Devrome H (2003) Consent for clinical research in the neonatal intensive care unit: a retrospective survey and a prospective study. *Arch Dis Child* **88**(4): F280–286

Cassileth BR, Lusk EJ, Miller DS, Hurwitz S (1982) Attitudes toward clinical trials among patients and the public. *JAMA* **248**: 968–70

Cox K (1999) Researching research: patients' experiences of participation in phase I and II anti-cancer drug trials. *Eur J Oncol Nurs* **3**: 143–52

Cox K (2000) Enhancing cancer clinical trial management: recommendations from a qualitative study of trial participants' experiences. *Psycho-oncology* **9**: 314–22

Cox K, McGarry J (2003) Why patients don't take part in cancer clinical trials: an overview of the literature. *Eur J Cancer Care* **12**(2): 114

Chalmers I (1998) Unbiased, relevant, and reliable assessments in health care. *Br Med J* **317**(7167): 1167–68

Dobkin BH (1990) A testing time: a doctor's thoughts on having his patients participate in double blind study of ticlopidine. *Discover* **11**: 86

Donovan JL, Mills N, Smith M, Brindle L, Jacoby A, Peters TJ *et al* (2002) Quality improvement report: improving design and conduct of randomised trials by embedding them in qualitative research: protect (prostate testing for cancer and treatment study). *Br Med J* **325**: 766–70

Dorantes DM, Tait AR and Naughton NN (2000) Informed consent for obstetric anesthesia research: factors that influence parturients' decisions to participate. *Anesth Analg* **91**(2): 369–73

Edwards SJL, Lilford RJ, Braunholtz, DA, Jackson J,C, Hewison J, Thornton J (1998) Ethical issues in the design and conduct of randomised controlled trials. *Health Technology Assessment* **2**(15)

Ellis PM (2000) Attitudes towards and participation in randomised clinical trials in oncology: a review of the literature. *Ann Oncol* **11**(8): 939–45

Featherstone K, Donovan JL (1998) Random allocation or allocation at random? Patients' perspectives of participation in a randomised controlled trial. *Br Med J* **317**(7167): 1177–80

Featherstone K, Donovan JL (2002) 'Why don't they just tell me straight, why allocate it?' The struggle to make sense of participating in a randomised controlled trial. *Soc Sci Med* **55**: 709–19

Ferguson PR (2002) Patients' perceptions of information provided in clinical trials. *J Med Ethics* **28**(1): 45–8

Field D *et al* on behalf of the INNOVO Trial Collaborating Group. Neonatal ventilation with INhaled Nitric Oxide versus Ventilatory support withOut inhaled nitric oxide for preterm infants with severe respiratory failure: The INNOVO multicentre randomised controlled trial (submitted)

Glogowska M, Campbell R, Peters TJ, Roulstone S, Enderby P. (2002) A multimethod approach to the evaluation of community preschool speech and language therapy provision. *Child Care, Health and Development* **28**(6): 513

Glogowska M, Roulstone S, Enderby P, Peters T, Campbell R (2001) Who's afraid of the randomised controlled trial? Parents' views of an SLT research study. *Int J Language Communication Disorders* **36**(suppl): 499–504

Gray BH (1975) *Human Subjects in Medical Experimentation: a sociological study of the conduct and regulation of clinical research*. Wiley, New York

Hassar M, Weintraub M (1976) Uninformed consent and the wealthy volunteer: an analysis of patient volunteers in a clinical trial of a new anti-inflammatory drug. *Clin Pharmacol Ther* **20**: 379–84

Henzlova MJ, Blackburn BH, Bradley EJ, Rogers WJ (1994). Patient perception of a long-term clinical trial: experience using a close-out questionnaire in the Studies of Left Ventricular Dysfunction (SOLVD) Trial. *Controlled Clinical Trials* **15**: 284–93

Howard JM, DeMets D (1981) How informed is informed consent? BHAT experience. *J Controlled Clinical Trials* **2**: 287–303

Jenkins V, Fallowfield L (2000) Reasons for accepting or declining to participate in randomised clinical trials for cancer therapy. *Br J Cancer* **82**(11):1783–8

Jones R (1995) Why do qualitative research? *Br Med J* **311**: 2

Kelle U (2001) Sociological explanations between micro and macro and the integration of qualitative and quantitative methods, forum. *Qualitative Research* **2**(1) http://www.qualitative-research.net/fqs-texte/1-01/1-01kelle-e.htm

Kemp N, Skinner E, Toms J (1984) Randomizad clinical trials of cancer treatment – a public opinion survey. *J Clin Oncol* **10**: 155–61

Kenyon SL, Taylow DW, Tarnow-Mordi W (2001a) Broad spectrum antibiotics for spontaneous preterm, prelabour rupture of fetal membranes: the ORACLE I trial. *The Lancet* **357**: 979–88

Kenyon SL, Taylor DJ, Tarnow-Mordi W (2001b) Broad spectrum antibiotics for spontaneous preterm labour: the ORACLE II randomized trial. *The Lancet* **357**: 989–94

Klein MC, Kaczorowski J, Robbins JM, Gauthier RJ, Jorgensen SH and Joshi AK (1995) Physicians' beliefs and behaviour during a randomized controlled trial of episiotomy: consequences for women in their care. *Can Med Assoc J* **156**(6): 769–78

Llewellyn-Thomas HA, McGreal MJ, Thiel EC, Fine S, Erlichman C (1991) Patients' willingness to enter clinical trials: measuring the association with perceived benefit and preference for decision participation. *Soc Sci Med* **32**(1): 35–42

Manning D (2000) Presumed consent in emergency neonatal research. *J Med Ethics* **26**: 249–53

Mason SA, Allmark PJ, Megone C, *et al* on behalf of the Euricon Study Group (2000) Obtaining informed consent to neonatal randomised controlled trials: interviews with parents and clinicians in the Euricon study. *The Lancet* **356**: 9247

Mettlin C, Cummings KM, Walsh D (1985) Risk factor and behavioural correlates of willingness to participate in cancer prevention trials. *Nutr Cancer* **7**(4): 189–98

Mills N, Donovan JL, Smith M, Jacoby A, Neal DE, Hamdy FC (2003) Patients' perceptions of equipoise are crucial to trial participation: a qualitative study of men in the ProtecT study. *Controlled Clinical Trials* **24**

Mohanna K, Tunna K (1999) Withholding consent to participate in clinical trials: decisions of pregnant women. *Br J Obstet Gynaecol* **106**(9): 892–7

Murray BL (2003) Qualitative research interviews: therapeutic benefits for the participants. *J Psychiatr Ment Health Nurs* **10**(2): 233-6

Muir Gray JA (1999) Postmodern Medicine. *The Lancet* **354**: 1550–3

Oakley A (1992) *Social Support and Motherhood*. Blackwell, Oxford

Oakley A (1998) Living in two worlds. *Br Med J* **316**: 482–83 (7 February)

Oakley A (2000) *Experiments in knowing: Gender and method in the social sciences*. Polity Press, Cambridge

Penman DT, Holland JC, Bahna GF and Morrow G *et al* (1984) Informed consent for investigational chemotherapy: patients and physicians' perceptions. *J Clin Oncol* **2**: 849–55

Pope C, Mays N (1995ii) Qualitative Research: Reaching the parts other methods cannot reach: an introduction to qualitative methods in health and health services research. *Br Med J* **311**: 42–5 (1 July)

Pope C, Mays N (1995i) Qualitative research: rigour and qualitative research. *Br Med J* **311**: 109–12 (8 July)

Ross S, Grant A, Counsell C, Gillespie W, Russell I, Prescott R (1999) Barriers to participation in randomised controlled trials: a systematic review. *J Clin Epidemiol* **52**: 1143–56

Ryan L (1995) Going public and watching sick people — the clinic setting as a factor in the experiences of gay men participating in AIDS clinical trials. *AIDS Care* **7**: 147–58

Salomons TV, Wowk AA, Fanning A, Chan VW, Katz J (2002) Factors associated with refusal to enter a clinical trial: epidural anesthesia is a deterrent to participation. *Can J Anaesth* **49**(6): 583–7

Saurbrey N, Jenson J, Elmegaard Rasmussen P, Gjorup T, Guldager H, Riis P (1984) Danish patients' attitudes to scientific-ethical questions. An interview study focusing therapeutic trials. *Acta Med Scand* **215**(2): 99–104

Smith P, Arnesen H (1988) Non-respondents in a post-myocardial infarction trial: characteristics and reasons for refusal. *Acta Med Scand* **223**(6): 537–42

Snowdon C, Garcia J, Elbourne D (1997) Making sense of randomization: responses of parents of critically ill babies to random allocation of treatment in a clinical trial. *Soc Sci Med* **45**: 1337–55

Snowdon C, Garcia J, Elbourne D (1998) Reactions of participants to the results of a randomised controlled trial: exploratory study. *Br Med J* **317**: 21–6

Snowdon C, Elbourne D, Garcia J (1999) Zelen randomization: attitudes of parents participating in a neonatal clinical trial. *Controlled Clinical Trials* **20**(2): 149–71

Snowdon C, Elbourne D, Garcia J (unpublished) Preliminary report of the study of parental and professional views of ECMO and hypothermia at Glenfield Hospital

Snowdon C, Elbourne D, Garcia J (in press) Perinatal pathology in the context of a clinical trial — attitudes of bereaved parents. *Arch Dis Child*

Sugarman J, McCrory DC, Powell D, Krasny A, Adams B, Ball E, Cassell C (1999) Empirical research on informed consent. An annotated bibliography. *Hastings Centre Report* **29**(1): S1–42

Tait AR, Voepel-Lewis T, Siewert M, Malviya S (1998) Factors that influence parents' decisions to consent to their child's participation in clinical anesthesia research. *Anesth Analg* **86**(1): 50–3

Tashakkori A, Teddle C (1998) *Mixed methdology: Combining qualitative and quanitative approaches*. Sage, London

Taylor KM, Margolese RG and Soskolne CL (1984) Physicians' reasons for not entering eligible patients in a randomized clinical trial of surgery for breast cancer. *N Engl J Med* **310**: 1363–67

Taylor KM, Feldstein ML, Skeel RT, Pandya KJ, Ng P, Carbone PP (1994) Fundamental dilemmas of the randomized clinical trial process: results of a survey of the 1,737 Eastern Cooperative Oncology Group investigators. *J Clin Oncol* **12**: 1796–1805

Tognoni G, Alli C, Avanzini F, Bettelli G, Colombo F, Corso R *et al* (1991) Randomised clinical trials in general practice: lessons from a failure. *Br Med J* **303**: 969–971

UK Collaborative ECMO Trial Group (1996) UK collaborative randomised trial of neonatal extracorporeal membrane oxygenation. *The Lancet* **348**: 75-82 (July 13th)

van Bergen PF, Jonker JJ, Molhoek GP, van der Burgh PH, van Domburg RT, Deckers JW, Hofman A (1995) Characteristics and prognosis of non-participants of a multi-centre trial of long-term anticoagulant treatment after myocardial infarction. *Int J Cardiol* **49**(2): 135–41

van Stuijvenberg M, Suur MH, de Vos S, Tjiang GCH, Steyerberg EW, Derksen-Lubsen G *et al* (1998) Informed consent, parental awareness, and reasons for participating in a randomised controlled study. *Arch Dis Child* **79**(2): 120–5

Walterspiel JN (1990) Informed consent: influence on patient selection among critically ill premature infants. *Pediatrics* **85**: 119–21

Williams RM, Thorn MH, Studd JWW (1980) A study of the benefits and acceptability of ambulation in spontaneous labour. *Br J Obstet Gynaecol* **87**: 122–26

Chapter 8

Exploring the healthcare experiences of people in hard to reach groups

Yana Richens and Lynne Currie

What matters more… is not being disadvantaged by poverty, race or disability,
but by the attitudes and reactions of those involved in care.

Hunt, 2003

Introduction

The purpose of this chapter is to provide insight on how the healthcare experiences of people who are traditionally labelled as 'hard to reach' can be explored by using qualitative or naturalistic research methodology. The chapter provides the reader with some ideas about the ways in which hard to reach groups can be involved in research. A qualitative study conducted by the first author will be offered as a detailed example of how focus-group method was used to explore the experiences of women of Pakistani origin who had used maternity services in England. In highlighting the challenges that may arise when attempting to explore the views of people from hard to reach groups, we list some of the potential pitfalls that researchers need to be aware of and plan for. We propose that focus-group method could be used in similar circumstances by groups of midwives and others involved in the care of people from hard to reach groups.

Which groups are 'hard to reach'?

People identified as 'hard to reach' are people who belong to a group which is outside the mainstream of society, and such people can be said to belong to marginalised groups. However, it is misleading to assume that people in hard to reach groups always live in poverty. Furthermore, a clear distinction needs to be made when we are considering hard to reach groups in relation to equalities in healthcare. While it may be argued that people who experience inequalities in terms of access to services, care and treatment include people from black and ethnic minority groups and asylum seekers, pregnant teenagers can also be included. As such, midwives should remain conscious of the way in which people from hard to reach groups are often stereotyped. For example, many black and ethnic minority women do speak English and many of them do not live in areas of high unemployment. In the same way, not all pregnant teenagers come from broken homes. However, many ethnic minority and black women are assumed to be non-English-speaking and living in poverty, while many pregnant teenagers continue to be labelled as coming from broken homes. We believe that all health professionals — not just midwives — must look beyond such stereotypes, must look beyond the 'labels' that are used to define people, and must start to see the real person behind the label. In addition to ethnic minority women, black women and pregnant teenagers, there are many people who belong to other groups that have been identified as being hard to reach — see *Box 8.1*.

Box 8.1: Examples of hard to reach groups (this list is not exhaustive)

❖ The homeless
❖ Asylum seekers
❖ Black and ethnic minorities
❖ Travellers
❖ Refugees
❖ Drug users
❖ Non-English-speaking people
❖ People who have English as a second language
❖ Victims of domestic violence
❖ Victims of sexual abuse
❖ Prisoners
❖ Pregnant teenagers
❖ People who are HIV-positive
❖ People with disabilities
❖ People with special needs

In terms of healthcare, people from hard to reach groups are often powerless and are unlikely to be provided with any opportunities to be involved or consulted on how health policies are set or how services are developed and delivered. Neither are they likely to be involved in research aimed at evaluating services. Actively involving and consulting hard to reach groups will only be achieved by being inclusive, by empowering people, and by overcoming marginalisation (Steel, 2001). People who belong to hard to reach or marginalised groups are said to be outside the dominant culture. The dominant culture may be a professional group or society as a whole. Whilst some people may be marginalised out of personal choice, more often than not they are marginalised because the dominant culture is unable or unwilling to accommodate them.

Accessing hard to reach groups in order to involve them in research requires tenacity and a proactive approach on the part of researchers. The best way to do this, according to Steel (2001), is through the use of local networks. He also argues that how difficult these groups are to reach depends on how hard we are prepared to try. Steel suggests several ways forward in reaching marginalised groups, including local councils, community voluntary services, local libraries, community centres, local gatherings, and word-of-mouth networking (*Box 8.2*).

Box 8.2: Ideas and recommendations for reaching marginalised groups

❖ Reaching marginalised groups will take time and careful thought
❖ Tapping into existing community networks, both formal and informal is often effective if done with sensitivity and respect
❖ Be aware that marginalised groups may not use the methods of communication you are used to
❖ Offer to meet people informally on their own ground and take time to build trust
❖ Be open and learn from them

Source: Steel R (2001) Involving Marginalised and Vulnerable Groups in Research: A Consultation Document

---

Accessing peoples' experiences of healthcare is a central tenet of the Government's policy on modernising the National Health Service (NHS), and this is clearly articulated in a range of policy documents (DoH, 1997; 1998; 2000; 2002a; 2002b). In addition, placing the patients' experience at the heart of health care is one of the five key elements of clinical governance, which is the Government's strategy for raising quality across the National Health Service (RCN, 2003).

Why use qualitative research to explore the experiences of hard to reach groups?

Evidence suggests that health outcomes in some hard to reach groups are different when compared to mainstream groups (Confidential Enquiries into Maternal Deaths [CEMD], 2001; Confidential Enquiries into Sudden Deaths in Infants [CESDI], 2001). However, such evidence is generally of a quantitative, statistical nature. For example, in the case of a non-English-speaking woman who has experienced midwifery care, a successful outcome can be measured as an intact perineum, whereas a less than successful outcome can be measured as a third degree tear. We are not suggesting that measuring outcomes is not important, but a primary focus on measuring the outcomes of care neglects the importance surrounding the process of care. An over-reliance on outcomes can lead to a disassociation from process, with the real possibility that patients or clients may have good outcomes (like an intact perineum) despite experiencing poor care, whereas others may have poor outcomes (like a third degree tear) while experiencing excellent care. Outcomes-based research tells us nothing about how people experience healthcare.

A useful means of accessing information about peoples' experiences of health care is through the use of qualitative research methodology. The use of qualitative research is aimed at an understanding of human experiences and actions within a natural, social context. In qualitative research, there is no attempt at measurement or quantification; no attempt at establishing causation; and no attempt at testing theory. The findings from this type of research are not generalisable, predictive or indicative of proof. One of the key functions of qualitative research is to provide some insight, or sensitisation to a particular phenomenon that people may have previously been unaware of. Qualitative researchers enter the world of the participants and seek to describe that world.

Research on hard to reach groups

While it has not been possible to include a review of all the research on hard to reach groups, we describe a number of studies that have sought to give healthcare professionals some insight into experiences of people who have been marginalised. These studies have largely been of a qualitative nature, and based in a community setting.

One researcher who explored the views and experiences of South Asian women about accessing contraception services managed to recruit participants successfully using a range of strategies (Lowe *et al*, 2004). She gained access to women through contact with the providers of English-language classes, Asian mother and baby groups, and the women's sewing circles. Lowe describes the process of recruitment as time-intensive, and argues that it required a significant effort on the part of the researcher to gain both the trust of community leaders and the women she wished to recruit. Lowe's findings suggest that women often found it difficult to access contraception services because of a range of barriers, including paternalism, refusal to refer, refusing the woman's request for contraception, and the women's acceptance of poor treatment.

In a study exploring the views of asylum seekers and refugees in the UK, McLeish (2001) gained access to participants by convenience and snowball sampling, through refugee support groups and health professionals. The findings highlighted a number of issues that were important to participants. These included; accommodation, vouchers, safety maternity services, language, staff attitudes, racism and support.

In a study exploring maternity care, Duff (1999) gained access to Bangladeshi women through community workers from the study locality. These women invited their friends and relatives to discuss their views about and experiences of maternity care, and more women were recruited from English-language classes, and mother and toddler groups.

As part of a PhD, Chapple (1998) sought the views of South Asian women who suffered from menorrhagia to discover whether there were any problems that had not been identified by GPs. In recruiting women to her study, Chapple visited several women's organisations and left information sheets, reply slips and stamped addressed envelopes, so women did not have to identify themselves in public. In addition, women were asked to pass this information to other women they knew to be suffering from menorrhagia. The researcher also visited a family centre used by South Asian women and spent some time there gaining their trust. She also visited the local health promotion unit and enlisted the support of a South Asian link worker. Chapple highlights how the link worker's support was invaluable in recruiting more women to the study, reassuring the women that their identities and words would remain anonymous, and in arranging and being present at the interviews. Chapple reported how she felt that it would be very difficult to gain access to South Asian women for a study looking at menstruation and menstrual blood. She reports that Asian families tended 'to be the most closed and private of all social groups' (Bhopal, 1995; cited in Chapple, 1998: 86).

What Chapple found, however, was that the women who took part in her study were keen to help; welcoming; candid; and very open. Her findings reveal that women wanted more information because they felt that their GPs provided limited advice about alternative treatments, and some reported how their GPs felt they complained unnecessarily. In addition, some of the women reported a lack of interpreters, as well as their fears around making a complaint because they believed that any future care might be jeopardised.

Problems associated with communication, information and education have been identified as key issues in a number of studies that have included ethnic minority women (Clarke and Clayton, 1983; Currer, 1986; Thomas *et al*, 1991; Bowler, 1993; Garcia *et al*, 1999; Gissler *et al*, 1998; Bradby, 2001; Hirst and Hewison, 2001; Petrou *et al*, 2001; McLeish, 2002). Researchers have found that language, culture and the ethnic origin of women and their carers have an effect on communication (Currer, 1986; Bowler, 1993; McLeish, 2002). These findings from research on hard to reach groups reinforce the message that poor communication has been identified as endemic across the NHS and is a major cause for complaint across all groups accessing healthcare services (Ombudsman, 2002).

Researchers in Finland highlighted how the under-use of ante-natal care is linked to foreign nationality, social class and young age (Gissler *et al*, 1998). Women of Pakistani origin make 9.1% fewer ante-natal visits (Petrou *et al*, 2001). Some commentators have suggested that this happens because Asian women are non-compliant (McFadyen and MacVicar, 1982). However, this idea of non-compliance has been critiqued by others who argue that the reasons for booking late may be cultural (Currer, 1986; Dobson, 1988).

Using focus groups to explore the experiences of hard to reach groups

There are a number of ways in which qualitative researchers can explore the healthcare experiences of people from hard to reach groups. In the example provided below, the method used to explore Pakistani women's experiences of UK maternity services was focus groups. A focus group is an in-depth, open-ended group discussion that explores a specific set of issues on a predefined and limited topic (see *Chapter 5*). Focus groups are convened under the guidance of a facilitator (Howard *et al*, 1989), provide direct feedback, and can be used as a way of obtaining rich information within a particular social context. Focus-group method has been used to elicit people's experiences of disease and health services (Barbour and Kitzinger, 1999). A distinguishing feature of focus-group method is the use of interaction as part of the research data (Kitzinger, 1994). It is an interview technique, and participants are a homogenous group of people who are asked a series of questions. During the interview, the participants hear other people's responses to the questions and are allowed to make additional comments if they wish (Chui and Knight, 1999). The groups are not required to reach any kind of consensus. Focus groups can facilitate the identification of cultural values and have been identified as being useful when researching ethnic minority groups (Hennings *et al*, 1996; Duff, 1999; Wilkins Winslow *et al*, 2002).

An exploration of Pakistani women's experiences of UK maternity services

The rationale for undertaking such an exploration was supported by data from the Confidential Enquiry into Sudden Deaths in Infants report (CESDI, 2001). This report outlined regional differences in perinatal mortality, and identified the West Midlands as having the highest perinatal mortality rates in England (13.2%). In addition, the

5th Confidential Inquiry into Maternal Deaths (CEMD 2001) highlighted how Asian women experience a three-times-higher risk of maternal death when compared with white women. The West Midlands have a large ethnic minority population, which made it an ideal location for the study. What follows is a brief summary of the study; a full description can be found in Richens (2003).

The objectives of the study were to describe the women's experiences, place these experiences within the context of current health policy, and make suggestions on ways to improve the delivery of maternity services to this group of women. A qualitative approach was taken to collecting and analysing data because it provides participants with both the opportunity to raise issues that are important to them and to be involved in the evaluation process.

Ethical approval was sought and received, although the women participating in this study expressed some concern regarding the requirement to sign a consent form (which is a clear requirement of the ethical process that researchers are required to follow). Because of cultural differences, women of Pakistani origin were offended at the idea that their word was not good enough and they were asked to sign a piece of paper. Researchers need to be aware of any potential cultural differences and plan their informed consent procedures accordingly. They will need to outline these procedures when making a submission for ethical approval. As part of the requirement for ethical approval, informed consent was sought and received from participants. The participants were assured that their responses and identity would remain confidential.

A purposive sampling strategy was employed to recruit women to the study. All participants had common characteristics in that they were women of Pakistani origin who had experienced UK maternity services on at least one occasion. No other factors (for example, age, marital status, method of delivery, incident of multiple births, language ability[1], place of birth, place of parent's birth) were used to exclude women. A pilot study was undertaken to test the focus-group interview schedule and to see how well the recruitment strategy worked. The key messages from the pilot study included making sure not to mix languages; revising the schedule to make it more general; and the recruitment of an Urdu-speaking research assistant.

The main focus groups were conducted in community and health centres and, on one occasion, a college. The venues for all the focus groups were based in the heart of the community where the women lived. This meant that women did not have to travel far or incur any heavy transport costs. Provision for children is also very important, and in this study one of the community centres provided a free crèche. However, during the majority of the focus-group discussions, the children played on the floor. Also, many of the women attended the meetings with their mothers-in-law or their sisters, and, while this is not an ideal research situation, researchers need to be aware of the cultural preferences of women from ethnic minorities. Being flexible in terms of meeting the requirements of the participants can result in a more successful recruitment strategy. A wider cultural

1. Throughout this chapter we use the term 'non-English speaking women' which is used to define those women who appeared unable to speak English. However, it is worth noting that even when this was the case, some of the women did understand many English words. Researchers would be advised to remain aware at all times that women can and do comprehend what is being said, even if they choose not to respond, or are unable to speak English.

awareness of the preferences of the target population will also lead the researcher to plan for the possibility that children and family members will attend, thereby ensuring that venues have plenty of space, and, even, enough food and drink for everyone.

Discussion

The challenges the researcher faced in gaining backing for the study were linked to gaining organisational support, recruiting the women, and collecting the data. The importance of speaking individually to the right gatekeepers about the research cannot be overestimated. Where a researcher is able to establish and sustain a trusting relationship with gatekeepers, one that is premised on a two-way process of communication, this can be a key success factor in gaining access to the research participants. It may also provide gatekeepers with a sense of ownership of the project.

While the provision of written information was a useful strategy, it was no substitute for talking to people. GPs who were known to have a high number of Pakistani women on their register were contacted. This was deemed important because GPs are the first point of contact for women who suspect that they may be pregnant. The researcher hoped that GPs would identify potential participants and allow access to the practice in order to recruit the women personally. However, despite a follow-up telephone call one month after sending the initial letter, this strategy proved unsuccessful. On reflection, it would have been more effective to have met with the practice midwife and health visitor. Hindsight also brought with it recognition of the important role of the GP's receptionist, another potential gatekeeper and a role that should never be underestimated.

Researchers also need to be aware of the sensitivities involved in seeking to access the views of ethnic-minority groups. While there was the potential to show that women of Pakistani origin may have positive experiences and feel fully supportive of midwifery services, they may also report negative experiences and highlight deficiencies in the service. This can often place the researcher in a very difficult position, especially when writing the report and making recommendations.

Prior to undertaking the study, the researcher met with a number of professionals working in the trust and interpreters working for the translation service. The purpose of the meeting was to provide an overview of the research, obtain gate-keeper support, and seek practical advice on recruitment. Prior to this meeting taking place, posters advertising the meeting were designed and circulated to all outreach clinics. This meeting was successful in gaining support and commitment from interpreters. Such success may be linked to the fact that the majority of interpreters lived in the Asian community, had strong links and contacts within the Asian community, and were committed to the aims of the study.

During the meeting, thought-provoking insights of those working for the translation service were shared, and while this data was not included for the purpose of analysis, it nevertheless provided the researcher with some very useful contextual information. It is advisable that researchers keep a clear set of field notes and meeting notes, since these are very useful when analysing data. What was clear from the views expressed by the interpreters during this meeting was that they did not feel valued; nor were they seen as part of the clinical team. This justifies the importance of actively targeting and gaining the support of the interpretation and translation service. The service can be a very real source of support for researchers who are seeking to explore the views of marginalised groups. There are, however, inconsistencies and confusion surrounding the role, function and definition of interpreters, translators, link workers and advocates. These terms are defined below:

⌘ An interpreter/translator facilitates communication between two people or groups of people by providing a literal translation of one language into another.
⌘ A link worker (generally employed by the NHS Trust) interprets and offers advice about cultural and religious issues, and acts as a link between staff and patients.
⌘ A bilingual advocate acts as an interpreter, and empowers users by ensuring they have access to information/services they may be unaware of (White *et al*, 1999).

Community leaders are an extremely valuable resource in the recruitment of women, who, in this case, were not current users of the service. It is important to build relationships with community leaders. In this study, local colleges and community centres that held English-language classes for non-English-speaking women were targeted and contacted by telephone. One centre was visited on three separate occasions, which helped establish a basis of trust between the researcher and the centre staff. These informal meetings were a useful way of enabling the staff to exchange information about the cultural context and the history of the centre, which serves several important functions in a multicultural part of the city. Exchanging information this way further supports the arguments made by Steel (2001) that being open and meeting people informally on their own ground is a very useful strategy, and that tapping into existing community networks can be very effective.

The challenges surrounding the recruitment of research participants can be considerable, and should never be underestimated. However, these challenges do not necessarily stem from potential participants being 'hard to reach'. What often slows down the recruitment of research participants are the processes that many researchers have to follow. For example, researchers are expected to write to trusts, consultants and GPs to get permission to access patients, and navigating a route through gatekeepers can be difficult. Since the purpose was to access women who were no longer patients, clients or users of the service, it was not necessary to go through the usual channels. All the women participating in the study were recruited through the community leaders, interpreters and the Urdu-speaking research assistant. Researchers need to be more creative and innovative when planning effective access strategies. We may, for example, need to consider in more detail gaining access to research participants through local radio, local newspapers, newsletters and shops, internet sources and support groups, in addition to those avenues suggested by commentators like Steel (2001).

It is also important to remember that interpreters do not always remain 'invisible' during the data collection process, as discovered in one of the focus group. On one occasion, the interpreter took it upon herself to ask probing questions, even when a participant had responded 'okay' to a question. On asking the woman additional probing questions, the interpreter was able to get the woman to reveal that in her experience, things had not really been 'okay' at all. Something similar to what we identify here as 'advocacy probing' has been reported by Hennings *et al* (1996). These commentators reported how an interpreter gently reminded a participant that she could feel free to tell the researcher what really happened by reassuring her that all responses, and her identity, would remain confidential (p. 17).

In terms of formalising the process of 'advocacy probing', one could speculate that researchers should make better use of interpreters' skills, knowledge and experience of talking with women from ethnic-minority groups in order to explore participants' experiences in greater depth. There is no reason why interpreters could not be seen as advocates for research participants, since their skills, knowledge and experience may result in them being much more adept at recognising any hesitation or reluctance in speaking out. As such, interpreters may be well-placed to ask gently probing questions in an attempt to elicit more information.

This process of 'advocacy probing' could be formalised through the use of terms of reference, which would be agreed between researcher and interpreter before data collection. The terms of reference would clearly articulate what the level of probing should be, and would also stipulate that leading questions should not be asked. Also important would be to ensure that the interpreter kept the researcher informed at all times during probing, thus allowing the researcher to interject and ask their own probing questions if appropriate. There is clearly a requirement for terms of reference to be agreed between the research team and the translation service when undertaking research on ethnic-minority groups, since researchers and interpreters are inextricably part of an inter-dependent relationship.

It is also crucial to understand that when undertaking focus groups with women whose first language is not English, extra time will be required. This is necessary because the interpreter needs to be given enough time to listen to the researcher's question, interpret this for the participants, check that it has been understood, listen to the response, and then interpret the responses for the researcher.

What may happen during focus groups is that women who speak English respond immediately, and also attempt to interpret the responses of the women who speak Urdu. While this did not really cause any great problems, it did require constant vigilance on the part of the researcher to ensure that all voices were heard. However, it is not possible to say with any certainty that the women who did not speak English did not comprehend some of what was being said, since it was apparent that they did have some understanding of spoken English. At the conclusion of each meeting, it appeared that women valued the opportunity to talk, so it may be beneficial for researchers to set aside some time at the end of the focus groups for this purpose. This informal talk can also provide opportunities to gain a broader understanding of both the cultural and local issues that are important to research participants. In this study, it was also useful in terms of recruitment, since many of the women recommended friends as potential participants at future meetings.

The research participants were extremely interested in knowing about the researcher. They also demonstrated a keen interest in midwifery and how to become a midwife. Such sharing of information helped to put both the participants and the researcher at ease, and enabled the building of relationships based on trust and a certain level of rapport. This is a very important message for researchers: they must be prepared to spend some time talking with participants once they have finished the data collection.

The study described above is an example of how a group of women whose views are not normally actively sought were successfully elicited. While this particular hard to reach group were women of Pakistani origin, we suggest that the key points and techniques described are relevant for researchers who are seeking to undertake research on a range of hard to reach groups.

Conclusion

In conclusion, we believe that the use of focus groups is a useful method in qualitative research to explore the experiences of people who belong to hard to reach groups. We also believe that this method could be used informally with groups of women who are being discharged into the community following the birth of their baby. Informal focus-group discussions may offer midwives an alternative practical solution to patient-satisfaction surveys in accessing clients' views about the maternity services they have received. We propose that these discussions could take place on a monthly basis, convened on the ward, with the hospital interpreter available to act as a translator. The discussions could be facilitated by clinical governance support staff, audit staff, or a midwife.

The information collected as a result of informal focus-group discussions would provide staff with an opportunity continuously to improve practice. Feeding back information to staff on the ward could be a powerful mechanism in providing staff with positive reinforcement, whilst also allowing staff the opportunity to get involved in identifying and solving any problems that may be highlighted. Furthermore, such a strategy clearly meets the requirements laid out in the *NHS Plan* (DoH, 2000) and in the *Framework for Clinical Governance* (RCN, 2003), which require all trusts to obtain feedback from patients about their experiences of care (DoH, 2000).

We have described the tendency to stereotype certain groups of people as being 'hard to reach', and have outlined several studies that have successfully elicited the views of people from hard to reach groups. We would suggest that such groups of people are not necessarily hard to reach: it is simply a matter of researchers thinking creatively about more effective routes of access and recruitment. As researchers, we need to be more innovative in thinking about what types of strategy we need to use to ensure that groups which in the past have been marginalised — and, in some cases, continue to be so — are provided with opportunities to participate in research. Furthermore, we need to ensure that these messages are translated in ways that reach midwives, obstetricians, policy-makers, research funders and politicians.

The success in recruiting Pakistani women to the study described above was facilitated greatly by going out into the community where Pakistani women lived and worked, and by building local networks based on mutual trust, respect and openness. We would like to end with an aphorism: where there's a will, there's a way.

References

Barbour RS, Kitzinger J, eds (1999) *Developing Focus Group Research — Politics, Theory and Practice*. Sage, London

Bradby H (2001) Communication, interpretation and translation. In: Culley L, Dyson S, eds. *Ethnicity and Nursing Practice*. Palgrave, Basingstoke

Bowler I (1993) They're not the same as us: midwives' stereotypes of South Asian women. *Sociol Health Illness* **81**(1): 46-65

Confidential Enquiries into Maternal Deaths (CEMD) (2001) *Why Mothers Die 1994–1996: Report on Confidential Enquiries into Maternal Deaths in the United Kingdom.* RCOG Press, London

Confidential Enquiries into Sudden Deaths in Infants (CESDI) (2001) *5th Annual Report.* London Maternal and Child Health Research Consortium

Chapple A (1998) Interviewing women from an ethnic minority group: finding the sample, negotiating access and conducting semi-structured interviews. *Nurs Standard* **6**(1): 85–92

Chui LF, Knight D (1999) How useful are focus groups for obtaining the views of minority groups? In: Barbour R, Kitzinger J (1999) *Developing Focus Group Research — Politics and Practice.* Sage, London

Clarke M, Clayton D (1983) Quality of obstetric care provided for Asian immigrants in Leicester. *BMJ* **297**: 384–7

Currer C (1986) *Health Concepts and Illness Behaviour: the Case of Some Pathan Mothers in Britain.* PhD thesis, University of Warwick

Department of Health (1997) *The New NHS: Modern, Dependable.* Stationery Office, London

Department of Health (1998) *A First Class Service: Quality in the New NHS.* Stationery Office, London

Department of Heath (2000) *The NHS Plan: a Plan for Investment, a Plan for Reform.* Stationery Office, London

Department of Health (2002a) *NHS Trust-Based Patient Surveys: Inpatients — Acute Hospitals.* Stationery Office, London

Department of Health (2002b) Partnership Working. Available online at: http://www.doh.gov.uk/prcare/pdfs/nsf_partnershipworking

Dobson S (1986) Ethnic Identity: a basis for care. *Midwife Health Visit Community Nurs* **24**(5): 172

Duff L (1999) *Development of an Interview Questionnaire to Measure Satisfaction with Maternity Care in Women from the Bangladeshi Community in England.* PhD thesis, London School of Hygiene and Tropical Medicine, University of London

Garcia J, Redshaw M, Fitzsimons B, Keene J (1998) *First Class Delivery: a National Survey of Women's Views of Maternity Care.* Audit Commission, Belmont Press, Northampton

Gissler M, Woolett M, Geraedts M, Hemminki E, Buekeris P (1998) Insufficient prenatal care in Finland and Baden. *Wurttemberg Eur J Pub Health* **8**: 227–31

Hennings J, Williams J, Naher, Haque B (1996) Exploring the health needs of Bangladeshi women: a case study in using qualitative research methods. *Health Educ J* **55**: 11–23

Hirst J, Hewison J (2001) Pakistani and indigenous white women's views and the Donabedian Maxwell grid: a consumer-focused template for assessing the quality of maternity care. *Int J Health Care Qual Assur* **14**(7): 308–16

Howard E, Huble Bank J, Moore P (1989) Employer evaluation of graduates: use of the focus group. *Nurs Educator* **14**(5): 38–41

Hunt S C (2003) *Poverty, Pregnancy and the Health Care Professional.* Elsevier, London

Katbamna S (2000) *Race and Childbirth.* Open University Press, Buckingham

Kitzinger J (1994) The methodology of focus groups: the importance of interaction between participants. *Sociol Health Illness* **16**: 103–21

Lowe P, Griffiths F, Siddhu R (2004) A consideration of institutional values preventing South Asian women accessing contraceptive services. A presentation at the Institute of Health, Walsgrave Hospital Seminar series: 28 January

McFayden I R, MacVicar J (1982) Obstetric problems of the Asian community in Britain. RCOG, London

McLeish J (2002) *Mothers in Exile — Maternity Experiences of Asylum Seekers in England.* The Maternity Alliance

Ombdusman (2002) *The Parliamentary Ombudsman: Annual Report.* Stationery Office, London

Petrou S, Kupek K, Vause S, Maresh M (2001) Clinical, provider and socio-demographic determinants of the number of antenatal visits in England and Wales. *Soc Sci Med* **52**: 1123–34

Richens Y (2003) Exploring the experiences of women of Pakistani origin of UK maternity services. Available online at: http://www.yanarichens.com

Royal College of Nursing (2003) *Clinical Governance: A Resource Guide.* RCN, London

Steel R (2001) Involving marginalised and vulnerable groups in research: a consultation document. Available online at: http://www.invo.org.uk/pub.htm. Accessed 9 October, 2003.

Thomas P, Golding J, Peters T J (1991) Delayed antenatal care: does it affect pregnancy outcome? *Soc Sci Med* **32**: 714–23

White P, Philips K, Minns A (1999) Women from ethnic minority communities: their knowledge of and needs for health advocacy services in east London. Staffordshire Press, Stoke-on-Trent

Wilkins WW, Honenin G, Elzubeir MA (2002) Seeking Emirati women's voices: the use of focus groups with an Arab population. *Qualit Health Res* **12**(4): 566–75

Chapter 9

How do you assess qualitative research?

Helen Smith

> *There is absolutely nothing that is seen by two minds simultaneously.*
> Bertrand Russell, 1872–1970

Introduction

What distinguishes good quality research from bad? How can the design, methods and findings of one qualitative study be judged against another? This chapter will help you make sense of qualitative research and answer these questions. It outlines different perspectives on the appraisal of qualitative research; summarises available checklists and criteria for evaluating qualitative research; and offers guidance on what to look out for when assessing qualitative research in health care.

Why assess qualitative research?

Quality assurance in qualitative research is becoming more important as wider exposure in health services research has increased interest in qualitative methods among researchers from other traditions. Quality assurance is the process by which research can be assessed for validity, reliability, value and relevance. Increased interest in qualitative research has led to closer inspection of the quality and rigour of conduct and outcomes, and a corresponding proliferation of checklists and criteria to evaluate qualitative research (for example, Blaxter, 1996; Treloar, 2000; Critical Appraisal Skills Programme [CASP], 2002; Malterud, 2001). Standards to distinguish good quality research from bad are important for two reasons. First, if the results of qualitative research are to have impact, potential users — including policy makers, researchers, practitioners and patients — need to be confident that they can believe the findings. Second, for researchers to produce good quality qualitative research, they need guidance on acceptable methods and processes.

Inadequate reporting of methods and procedures of qualitative inquiry by qualitative researchers, commonly a result of limited space in non-specialist journals, is one reason for misunderstandings about qualitative inquiry and frequent criticism of 'inferior' methods from quantitative researchers (Bryman, 1988). The most common criticisms, according to Mays and Pope (1995), are that qualitative research is merely an assembly of anecdotal and personal impressions, strongly subject to researcher bias; that qualitative research lacks reproducibility (the research is so personal to the researcher that there is no guarantee that a different researcher would not come to radically different conclusions); and that there is poorer generalisability.

Qualitative researchers have confronted these criticisms in a variety of ways. Checklists and standards for assessing the quality of qualitative research have played an important part, particularly over the last decade. In healthcare research, the main challenge has been legitimising qualitative research among those who speak a different professional language. Elliot *et al* (1999) suggest that guidelines for qualitative research in clinical psychology are needed to 'help legitimise qualitative research, to foster more valid scientific reviews of qualitative research, and to improve the quality of research being conducted'. Leininger (1994) argues that the development of quality criteria for qualitative research are long overdue and, without them, 'we will continue to have non-credible, inaccurate, and questionable findings for qualitative studies'.

Others suggest that standards for qualitative research are important to counter the possibility of methodological supremacy in health-related research. For example, Popay *et al* (1998) note, 'in the absence of any attempt to develop standards, there is a danger that qualitative research evidence will be misunderstood and judged inferior by those whose field of vision is firmly fixed on a hierarchy of evidence that makes randomised controlled trials the gold standard'. Malterud (2001) also believes that enhancing the credibility of qualitative research through guidelines and standards can prevent methodological separatism in medical research:

> *Responsible application of qualitative research methods is a promising*
> *approach to broader understanding of clinical realities. No research method*
> *will ever be able to describe people's lives, minds and realities completely*
> *though, and medical doctors should be reminded that scientific knowledge is*
> *not always the most important or relevant type of information when dealing*
> *with people.*

Qualitative research now enjoys unprecedented popularity in the field of health research (Barbour, 2001). The dichotomy between qualitative and quantitative methods is less apparent, and both approaches are increasingly being used together to answer health services research questions. Qualitative methods are frequently used as a preliminary to quantitative research alongside quantitative research to validate or provide a different perspective on the phenomenon being studied, or independently to uncover processes and perspectives not accessible via traditional quantitative methods (see Pope and Mays, 2000). However, there remains widespread concern among qualitative researchers over ensuring quality and credibility in qualitative research (Spencer *et al*, 2003). As Barbour suggests (2001), 'the question is no longer whether qualitative methods are relevant, but how rigour can be ensured or enhanced'. Many checklists, guidelines and criteria for assessing qualitative research exist, developed by methodologists from different philosophical perspectives. This chapter provides an overview of the different perspectives on criteria to assess qualitative research, and summarises the key features of several published criteria developed within the health field.

Chapter outline

This chapter first outlines the general principles of assessing the quality of research. It then discusses different perspectives on criteria to assess the quality of qualitative research. Next it summarises a selection of published criteria and checklists and highlights some features that appear to be common across different criteria. Finally, it provides a practical guide to using criteria, with examples of what to look for when assessing qualitative research.

Assessing the quality of research

The basic strategy to ensure rigour in research, regardless of design, includes integrity and competence in planning and conducting research, and steps to limit the likelihood that bias will affect the collection, analysis and interpretation of data. One also has to ensure that the research is relevant and useful (Mays and Pope, 1995). Conventional criteria to judge quality are based on internal and external validity and reliability. This means a study should be able to demonstrate the extent to which data collection, analysis and interpretation are free from bias; that the findings are generalisable across different settings and populations; and that the findings are consistent with the data collected (Cook and Campbell, 1979). *Table 9.1* lists key criteria for judging quantitative research and an explanation of each.

Table 9.1: Criteria for judging quantitative research	
Criteria	**Interpretation**
Internal validity	Truth value or believability of the research findings
External validity	Whether the findings are applicable to other settings and populations
Reliability	The consistency of the findings
Objectivity	The absence of bias; neutrality in the research process

Qualitative researchers have repeatedly critiqued the assumptions of quantitative methods, claiming over-emphasis on control and objectivity, and lack of attention to context. However, in fervently pursuing criticisms of quantitative methods, Silverman (1989) suggests that qualitative researchers have neglected to provide a comparable programme for qualitative research, or adequately define standards by which the methods can be judged. Many qualitative methodologists agree that while common elements exist, there is a general lack of consensus about the assumptions that underpin qualitative research. As Sandelowski (1986) points out, this has made it difficult to defend the methodological rigour of qualitative research:

> *The debate surrounding the methodological rigour of qualitative research is confounded by its diversity and lack of consensus about the rules to which it ought to conform and whether it is comparable to quantitative research.*

Growing interest in qualitative methods, wider exposure in health research, and the need for critical appraisal of qualitative studies to inform evidence-based practice has led to closer scrutiny of qualitative approaches (Popay *et al*, 1998; Dixon-Woods and Fitzpatrick, 2001). As researchers from other traditions begin to understand the methods, they are demanding a means by which they can evaluate the claims researchers make about the design, conduct and outcomes of qualitative research (Mays and Pope, 2000).

As a result, there has been a proliferation of frameworks, checklists and criteria for assessing qualitative research over the past ten years, with a high proportion of them developed in medical or health-services research.

Different perspectives on quality criteria for qualitative research

While most qualitative researchers agree the need for standards by which good research can be distinguished from bad, there are some who argue that the search for any criteria is fundamentally wrong (Murphy *et al*, 1998). These differing perspectives largely stem from the researcher's stance on the philosophical basis of qualitative research. The rejection of criteria altogether is associated with Smith (1984) and his assumption that qualitative research is based on an idealist philosophy. He argues that reality does not exist independently beyond individual human constructions. Therefore, a certain or correct understanding of reality is impossible, since there are as many realities as there are people (Smith, 1984; Spencer *et al*, 2003). Idealists believe that all research perspectives are unique, and each is equally valid in its own right (Mays and Pope, 2000). Attempting to define any criteria to evaluate the trustworthiness of different versions of reality is therefore unrealistic (Smith, 1984). Acceptance of Smith's argument and rejection of quality standards makes it impossible to judge the quality and relevance of one study over another.

Alternative views on the philosophical basis of qualitative research make it easier to accept the notion of criteria for assessing quality. Realists believe the world has an existence independent of our perception of it, and there is an underlying 'reality' that can be studied. Hammersley (1992) argued that no research method can objectively reproduce that reality, but it is possible to represent it by obtaining knowledge we are relatively confident about. Hammersley called this third position between idealism and realism 'subtle realism'. The subtle-realist approach opens up the possibility that research can produce multiple, non-competing, valid descriptions of the same phenomenon, and that these can be assessed against quality criteria common to qualitative and quantitative research (Murphy *et al*, 2003).

The lack of agreement about the philosophical basis, nature and practice of qualitative research has specific implications for the development of quality standards. Among those who agree that quality criteria can be identified and applied to qualitative research, there exists a range of views about the content and form they should take. In general, there are those who believe conventional criteria can be applied to qualitative research, and those who argue for alternative criteria specific to this type of research.

Alternative criteria for assessing qualitative research

The most common critique of the application of conventional criteria for scientific rigour in quantitative research to qualitative research is by Lincoln and Guba (1985). They argue that it is fundamentally inappropriate to apply criteria used to assess research from a positivist paradigm to research grounded in a naturalist paradigm. They took four criteria characteristic of a positivist or quantitative paradigm (internal validity, external validity, reliability and objectivity) and developed appropriate alternatives to assess the 'trustworthiness' of qualitative research. *Table 9.2* shows Lincoln and Guba's alternative criteria, which they admit correspond in some ways to validity and reliability in quantitative research, but focus on the nuances of a qualitative approach.

Table 9.2: Lincoln and Guba's alternative 'qualitative' criteria	
Qualitative term	**Interpretation**
Credibility (*internal validity*)	Whether or not the participants studied find the account true and believable
Transferability (*external validity*)	Whether findings are transferable to other settings, given adequate description of context
Dependability (*reliability*)	Whether all methods and decisions are documented in an audit trail
Confirmability (*objectivity*)	Whether the findings are grounded in the data
Italics denotes comparable criteria for assessing quantitative research Adapted from Lincoln and Guba (1985)	

Some authors avoid the use of quantitative criteria in their checklists. For example, in Beck's (1993) criteria to evaluate qualitative research in nursing, the quantitative terms internal validity, external validity and reliability are referred to as 'credibility, fittingness and auditability, respectively... which are more appropriate to qualitative research'. Leininger's (1994) criteria for evaluating qualitative research also build on the work of Guba and Lincoln, and emphasise the importance of credibility, confirmability, meaning-in-context, recurrent patterning, saturation and transferability . *Box 9.1* lists some questions that appear in checklists derived from Guba and Lincoln's 'alternative criteria'

Box 9.1: Questions to ask of a qualitative study — emphasis on 'trustworthiness'

❖ Is the research aiming to explore the subjective meanings that people give to particular experiences?
❖ Were the data collected in a way that addressed the research issue?
❖ Has the relationship between researcher and participants been adequately considered?
❖ Are different sources of knowledge about the issues being explored or compared?
❖ Do the researchers make explicit the process by which they move from data to interpretation.

Adapted from Popay *et al* (1998) and CASP (2001)

Conventional criteria for assessing qualitative research

Hammersley (1990), Le Compte and Goetz (1982) and Kirk and Miller (1986), among others, maintain that qualitative research can be assessed with the same broad criteria as quantitative research. They argue that the aim of qualitative research is to represent reality rather than reproduce it, and that there are ways to assess different perspectives presented by different research against each other. They support conventional approaches to assessing the quality of research and advocate the use of quality criteria common to both quantitative and qualitative research — in particular, validity, reliability and relevance. The terminology associated with this subtle-realist perspective is therefore closely aligned with that of quantitative (positivist) traditions. For example, criteria developed by Cobb and Hagemaster (1987) use concepts common to both quantitative and qualitative paradigms and suggest categories for evaluation that 'do not depart greatly from what might be found in any scientific proposal'. Mays and Pope (1995) believe validity and relevance are essential to good-quality qualitative research and suggest ways to improve both. To improve validity, they suggest using: i) triangulation (employing two or more methods of data collection); ii) respondent validation (comparing the investigators' account of findings with participants' accounts to establish correspondence between the two); and iii) clear detailing of data collection and analysis methods. To increase relevance, they suggest using sampling methods that ensure as wide a range of participants as possible, and propose that adequate explanatory theory and descriptive detail can help determine the generalisability of the findings. Both Blaxter (1996) and Treloar's (2000) criteria are intended for use with researchers from biomedical and clinical backgrounds. The criteria are based firmly on concepts of validity and reliability, and use terms familiar to quantitative researchers (Blaxter, 1996; Treloar, 2000). *Box 9.2* lists key questions that commonly appear in published checklists that use conventional criteria for assessing qualitative studies.

Box 9.2: *Questions to ask of a qualitative study: emphasis on validity and relevance*

❖ Is the purpose of the study clearly stated?
❖ Is an appropriate rationale provided for using a qualitative approach?
❖ Does the researcher address threats to the reliability and validity in data collection, analysis and interpretation?
❖ Have measures been taken to test the validity of the findings?
❖ What conclusions were drawn and are they justified by the results?

Adapted from Treloar (2000), Blaxter (1996), Greenhalgh and Taylor (1997)

Criteria for judging 'good practice' in qualitative research

The various perspectives on quality criteria make it difficult for qualitative researchers to agree on and communicate what constitutes good-quality research to other researchers, especially those from different scientific traditions. This section summarises a selection of published criteria and checklists, and highlights some features that appear to be common across different criteria. The list of criteria in *Table 9.3* is not exhaustive: a quick literature search will yield many more references to 'guidelines for appraising', 'checklists for evaluating' and 'criteria for assessing' qualitative research. This summary represents a selection of eight criteria developed specifically within the health, medical and nursing fields.

Table 9.3: Key features of selected criteria developed within the medical and nursing fields				
Authors	**Assumptions of criteria**	**Format**	**Purpose**	**Field**
Blaxter (1996)	Uses, concepts and language from quantitative paradigm, but emphasises differences in qualitative methods	20 questions addressing methods, analysis, context and ethics	Guidance for journal editors on evaluating qualitative papers; methods teaching; proposal writing	Medical sociology
Cobb and Hagemaster (1987)	Uses concepts common to quantitative and qualitative paradigms, but categories address concerns unique to qualitative research	Checklist of 10 criteria including: context; importance to nursing; ethics	Evaluating research proposals	Nursing
Greenhalgh and Taylor (1997)	Emphasises importance of ground rules for critical appraisal of qualitative research	Nine questions including: researcher's perspective; quality control in analysis; credibility and transferability	Evaluating papers that describe qualitative research	Medical
Leininger (1994)	Inappropriate to apply quantitative criteria to qualitative studies as truth value and meaning will be lost	Six criteria that focus on trustworthiness	Evaluating qualitative research papers	Nursing
Malterud (2001)	Underlying principles of research similar in both paradigms, importance of overall standards	Guidelines that focus on relevance, validity and reflexivity	Guidelines for authors and reviewers of qualitative studies	General medical
Mays and Pope (1995)	Qualitative research can be assessed using same broad criteria as quantitative	Key questions that focus on validity and relevance	Evaluating qualitative studies	Health

Treloar *et al* (2000)	A synthesis of guidelines for best practice in qualitative research; acceptance that appraisal of qualitative research requires different skills	Ten-point critical appraisal checklist focusing on rigour, generalisability and reflexivity	Critical appraisal of studies; guidance for designing and publishing qualitative research	Clinical epidemiology
QRHWG (2002)	Quality criteria for applied qualitative health research developed by a multidisciplinary team; need to obtain consensus on standards of rigour in qualitative methods	Six key questions with hints to help judge how well the research addresses each criteria	Assessing qualitative studies; methods teaching; evaluating proposals	Health

Although developed nine years later and within a different field, the criteria proposed by Blaxter (1996) are very similar to that of Cobb and Hagemaster (1987). They both state explicitly that while the evaluative categories and language used do not differ from those found within a quantitative framework, the content of each category addresses concerns unique to qualitative research. For example, they both contain questions that address the purpose of the study, allowing an assessment of the appropriateness of a qualitative approach. Both criteria also address the context of the study. The questions are whether the setting and subjects are adequately described; whether the researcher-respondent relationship is fully understood; and whether the role and influence of the researcher have been examined critically. Lastly, they both consider whether ethical issues have been adequately addressed — an important aspect of qualitative research that is overlooked by some other criteria.

The checklists proposed by Treloar *et al* (2000) and Greenhalgh and Taylor (1997) were developed specifically for the critical appraisal of published qualitative research and they share many common areas. Both emphasise the importance of ground rules for evaluating qualitative studies and aim to provide a framework for best practice in qualitative research. Both checklists were developed within the medical field, primarily as a result of the increasing popularity of qualitative methods in the biomedical sciences. They acknowledge that critical appraisal of published qualitative research requires different skills and tools to the conventions that exist for evaluating quantitative and epidemiological research. Greehalgh and Taylor (1997) emphasise the importance of validity, while Treloar *et al* (2000) argue that the qualities most appropriate for qualitative studies within epidemiology are rigour, generalisability and reflexivity.

Social scientists within the Qualitative Research in Health Working Group (QRHWG) at Liverpool School of Tropical Medicine (LSTM) have developed pragmatic criteria for assessing qualitative research that set broad standards for 'good practice' (QRHWG, 2002), something Miles and Huberman alluded to when they suggested, 'It is possible to develop practical standards — workable across different perspectives — for judging the goodness of conclusions...' (Miles and Huberman, 1994). The criteria represent a synthesis of several published checklists and guidelines and were developed by a multi-disciplinary team, comprising researchers and lecturers actively engaged in qualitative research in the health field. Team members represent different philosophical perspectives and disciplinary backgrounds, but agreed on the following assumptions prior to developing the criteria:

1. Most published criteria attribute importance to validity, reliability and generalisability, but the terminology used varies according to philosophical and methodological perspective. Clarity in language used to describe rigour in qualitative methods is essential for communicating with researchers from different backgrounds.
2. As applied health research becomes question — rather than theoretically — driven (the qualitative-quantitative divide is narrowing), there is a need to bridge the overstated gap between different philosophical stances within the qualitative research tradition in order to obtain consensus on standards of rigour in qualitative methods.
3. Researchers in any discipline can, and should, take steps to enhance the quality of the research process and outputs. Reasonable rules for 'good practice' in qualitative research methods exist, and should be made explicit.

The criteria were designed for use by individuals with differing levels of understanding of qualitative research. They can be used to assess qualitative research outputs, to guide inexperienced researchers in the design and conduct of qualitative research, and to remind more experienced researchers of ways to improve rigour at each stage. The criteria address all six key stages of the qualitative research process, beginning with the rationale and study design, moving through sampling and data collection to analysis, findings and interpretation, and implications.

The criteria summarised above and in *Table 9.3*, while not exhaustive, illustrate the range of options available for assessing qualitative research. Most authors do not claim comprehensiveness or universal applicability, but stress the need for further validation and modification of their criteria (Greenhalgh and Taylor, 1997; Malterud, 2001). Due to the very nature of qualitative research, the differing perspectives of researchers and the various applications of quality criteria, it is unlikely that one universally applicable checklist will ever emerge from the debate. The best advice for now would be to select a checklist or set of criteria that best fit your own perspective and are most appropriate for the task, be it critical appraisal of an individual paper, designing a study or evaluating a research proposal.

Practical guide to using criteria to assess qualitative research

This section provides examples of what to look for when using criteria to assess qualitative research, drawing on questions that are common to all the criteria summarised in *Table 9.3*. Illustrations of 'good practice' in qualitative research, extracted from relevant medical and midwifery literature are provided throughout.

Is the problem clearly defined with an appropriate rationale for using a qualitative approach?

A good qualitative study begins with a clearly thought-out question to address an important clinical problem or health issue (Greenhalgh and Taylor, 1997). Have a look back at *Chapter 2*, which outlines the foundations of qualitative enquiry, and how it differs from the rigid experimental nature of quantitative research. Qualitative research aims to answer 'what', 'how' and 'why' questions. Questions such as, 'what prevents TB patients from adhering to treatment?', 'how do women feel about having a continuous support person present throughout labour?' or 'why do young women decide to start smoking?' are best answered using carefully chosen qualitative data-collection methods. Recall that the strength of a qualitative approach is its ability to go beyond measuring the problem. The aim should be to understand the subjective experiences or views of those being researched. Indicators of a good study include a clearly defined research question and evidence that the researcher is confident about the purpose of the research.

Next, it is important to determine whether a qualitative approach is appropriate to answer the question, and if it is adequately justified. The methodology should clearly seek to understand what is happening, and the reasons for observed situations, outcomes or discourses. The example in *Box 9.2*, from a study of the use of evidence-based leaflets in maternity care (Stapleton, 2002), illustrates good practice in terms of defining the rationale for a qualitative study.

Box 9.2: Good practice for defining the rationale for a qualitative study

... ten research-based leaflets (Informed Choice) were developed by the Midwives and Information and Resource Service to support consumer choice. The effectiveness of these leaflets has been studied in a randomised controlled trial, which is reported separately. To understand the social context in which the leaflets were used we undertook qualitative research alongside, but independently of, the randomised controlled trial.

Attitudes of staff are thought to influence the choices available to childbearing women and decision-making in clinical practice. Organisational culture affects the quality of health care. Socially complex interventions, such as Informed Choice leaflets, should be evaluated within the context in which they are used and through a prudent combination of qualitative and quantitative methods.

Is the study design appropriate to the purpose and the research question?

When evaluating the design of a qualitative study, the most important points to clarify are whether the objectives are clearly defined, and if the methods used are appropriate to the research question. The design should be clearly linked to, and follow on from, the study rationale. The objectives should be consistent with the key assumptions of a qualitative approach: for example, to explore, interpret, explain or understand a particular issue.

The methods chosen should be appropriate to address the research question and objectives. Methods commonly used in qualitative research include interviewing (in-depth or semi-structured); focus group discussions; and observation and document analysis. Ask: would other (quantitative) methods address the issue better?

Triangulation is the use of multiple methods; multiple data sources, multiple methods for examining data, and multiple researchers of methods to improve the validity of the findings and to ensure they are not the product of a single method, a single source, or a single researcher's bias. If triangulation of methods is not specified, ask yourself whether use of a single method is justified.

The example in *Box 9.3*, extracted from a study of influences on smoking behaviour in Bangladeshi and Pakistani adults (Bush *et al*, 2003), illustrates good practice in defining study objectives and methods.

Box 9.3: Good practice in defining study objectives and methods

[The objective of this study was] to gain a detailed understanding of influences on smoking behaviour in Bangladeshi and Pakistani communities in the United Kingdom to inform the development of effective and culturally acceptable smoking cessation interventions.

[The design was] a qualitative study using community participatory methods, purposeful sampling, one to one interviews, focus groups, and a grounded theory approach to data generation and analysis.

Are the issues of sampling in qualitative research appropriately addressed?

Qualitative sampling techniques differ from randomised strategies used to select representative samples in clinical and epidemiological research. Qualitative studies usually employ non-probability or purposive sampling to select participants based on their experience of the issue being studied. In qualitative research, in-depth understanding is more important than representativeness. It is necessary to determine whether the participants selected will allow comparisons to test and generate theoretical ideas about that population. Qualitative researchers use various non-probability strategies, including convenience sampling, quota sampling and theoretical sampling. A good-quality study will describe in detail how participants were selected and why.

What methods of data collection are used and are the procedures clearly described?

Qualitative researchers are frequently criticised for inadequate reporting of methods. A good study will provide information about how data-collection procedures were developed, including topic guides and checklists for interviews and focus-group discussions, and details of any adjustments made to tools after pilot testing. The researcher should also demonstrate familiarity with key methodological references.

To determine the extent of researcher influence on the data-collection process, details of who conducted data collection should be documented along with an appreciation of their skills, motives and perspectives. There are no rules as to how much detail should be provided, but a simple guide is to ask yourself, 'Have I been given enough information about the selection of participants and the methods used?'

The example in *Box 9.4* is taken from a study to understand smoking in Bangladeshi and Pakistani adults (Bush *et al*, 2003), and illustrates good practice in sampling and data collection methods.

Box 9.4: Good practice in detailing sampling and data-collection methods

... community researchers held semi-structured interviews with thirty-seven participants and twenty-four focus groups (with 104 participants). Interviews and focus groups were based on topic guides, translated into relevant South Asian languages by the community researchers. Twenty pilot interviews and focus groups took place to give the researchers confidence, to test the feasibility of recruitment techniques, and to refine the topic guides.

Research participants were sampled purposively... on the basis of ethnic group, sex, age, smoking status and occupation. Both male and female smokers were recruited... informally through community-based religious and non-religious organizations and groups using a 'snowballing' technique — where a small number of informants put the researcher in touch with others, who then nominate friends, colleagues and other contacts.

Have ethical issues been adequately considered?

Given the in-depth nature of qualitative enquiry, an understanding of how the research might affect participants' rights and welfare is essential. In the context of UK health research, the *Research Governance Framework for Health and Social Care* defines the broad principles of good research governance, and helps ensure that research is conducted to high scientific and ethical standards (Department of Health, 2003). It outlines these standards and details the responsibilities of the key people involved in research. Adhering to these ethical principles can ensure the goals of the research are met, while maintaining the rights of the research participants.

Researchers should report whether the research was approved by an ethics committee and complied with local institutional requirements, and what methods were used to ensure confidentiality and privacy. Particularly important in qualitative research is negotiation of consent: participants should receive a detailed explanation of any possible benefits and risks associated with participation in the study, and the researcher should clarify the procedures used to obtain informed consent.

Are accepted methods of data analysis used and how systematic is the analysis?

Analysing the accumulation of narrative data from interviews and focus-group discussions is, for most qualitative researchers, the most challenging and time-consuming phase of a qualitative study. There are no hard and fast rules on how to analyse qualitative data, but it is generally accepted that sifting through the data for interesting quotations, or selecting extracts of narrative that support a particular theory, are unacceptable. The researcher must make reference to accepted procedures for analysis: for instance, the framework approach (Ritchie and Spencer, 1994), grounded theory (Glaser and Strauss, 1967), or content analysis (Bryman and Burgess, 1994). Whatever procedure is used, the researcher must be able to describe a systematic process that identifies not only recurring themes and categories derived from majority views, but examples that contradict or challenge emerging theories.

Some qualitative researchers employ computer software to help analyse text. Packages such as WinMAX (Kuckartz, 2002) and NUD*IST (Gahan and Hannibal, 1999) can support data handling, but it is important for the researcher to demonstrate an understanding of the limits of computer-aided analysis, and provide adequate description of how and why the software was used. A good qualitative researcher will provide enough detail so that an independent researcher could follow and replicate the process and arrive at similar conclusions.

Equally important in qualitative data analysis is attention to measures to enhance the reliability and validity of the process. Allowing more than one researcher to identify independently emerging themes, code transcripts and interpret the data can enhance the reliability (consistency) of data analysis by confirming that both are assigning the same meaning to the data. Respondent validation (feeding back findings to participants) and triangulation of data from different sources can improve the validity (believability) of the analysis process and the researcher's conclusions.

The example in *Box 9.5*, extracted from a qualitative and quantitative study examining the relationship between private health insurance and high Caesarean section rates in Chile (Murray, 2000), illustrates good practice in qualitative data analysis.

Box 9.5: Good practice in qualitative data analysis

The transcripts of the in-depth interviews were analysed by using QSR NUD*IST software to facilitate cross-indexing. The entire Spanish text was entered. I carried out the coding and analysis. I examined the transcripts closely for emerging themes and coded blocks of text into nine broad categories of statement generated from the data. I examined the data for evidence of 'negative instances' that might contradict these emerging themes, explored the reasons for these, and modified my interpretation accordingly. I used survey data and other institutional statistics to test the qualitative conclusions and to examine possible counter-explanations.

What conclusions are drawn, and are they justified by the data?

Determining the accuracy and relevance of qualitative research is not as straightforward as calculating confidence intervals or conducting significance tests. It is a case of assessing whether the results are reasonable and believable, and whether they actually contribute new knowledge and are important in the local context studied. Look for evidence that the researcher's claims are supported by actual data: for example, a general statement that 'most of the women interviewed were fearful of Caesarean section' requires two, if not more, verbatim quotations to illustrate the range of views on the issue. To ensure the results are verifiable, quotations should be indexed or labelled so they can be traced to a particular person and setting.

In qualitative research, it is often difficult to separate what the researchers found from what they think it means, because the results are in effect an interpretation of the data. It is necessary then to make a judgement on how coherent the findings are to what is already known, and how well the interpretation explains why people behave the way they do (Greenhalgh and Taylor, 1997). In addition, the researcher should avoid tainting the findings with his or her own personal or cultural perspectives. This is difficult to judge even if the researcher provides evidence of reflection on his or her own role, bias and influence on the research.

To determine the relevance and value of qualitative research requires making a judgement on whether the findings address the original research question, and whether they contribute new knowledge or understanding. Key points to look for include: a discussion that clearly links the findings to the aims and objectives of the study; discussion of how the findings contribute to existing knowledge and previous research; and whether the findings conceptualise new insights or alternative ideas about the phenomenon being studied.

Are the findings applicable in populations and settings other than the study context?

Qualitative research is frequently criticised for lacking external validity, or wider transferability. In other words, the findings and implications are perceived to be limited to the particular setting in which the research was conducted. If convenience sampling is used, the findings are more likely to apply only in the setting in which they were generated. However, Mays and Pope (2000) suggest that theoretical sampling — where an initial sample is selected to include as diverse a range of population characteristics as possible, but is modified to include others as theory emerges — can improve generalisability of findings. This strategy helps to ensure that the complete sample includes the full range of perspectives relevant to the subject, and makes it possible to test whether emerging findings are applicable to different participants.

If the researcher provides enough descriptive detail of the study setting, this can also help determine the applicability of the findings to other settings and populations. Indicators to look for in qualitative studies include adequate description of the local context (geographical, cultural, political, socio-economic) and a discussion of the scope for generalising findings to populations or settings other than the study sample.

The example in *Box 9.6*, taken from the study of influences on smoking in Bangladeshi and Pakistani adults (Bush *et al*, 2003), shows how the authors described the scope for generalisability of the study findings.

Box 9.6: Good practice in describing scope for generalisability

Although our results show some similarities with studies of smoking behaviour in predominantly white populations, they also highlight important differences... the findings must be interpreted with regard to the characteristics of our sample and the participatory nature of the research. We had a broad range of participants in terms of age, sex, occupation, socioeconomic status, education level and smoking status. By working with members of communities at all stages of the research, we used our participatory approach to increase the validity of our findings. The socioeconomic characteristics of Bangladeshi and Pakistani people living in Newcastle on Tyne are broadly typical of Bangladeshi and Pakistani people nationally. Thus, although we must be guarded, our findings are likely to be generalisable to other Bangladeshi and Pakistani communities in the United Kingdom, although local variations may exist.

Conclusions

Inexperienced qualitative researchers in the field of health care should be aware that there is much disagreement about how qualitative research should be planned, conducted and analysed, but should not be put off by the apparent lack of clarity on what constitutes 'good practice' (Chapple, 1998). Debate between researchers from different philosophical and methodological perspectives over the most appropriate criteria for assessing qualitative research will continue, and modifications to existing criteria and checklists are inevitable.

It is the author's opinion that it is possible to rise above the philosophical and methodological debate that surrounds criteria for assessing qualitative research. Reasonable rules for 'good practice' in qualitative research methods do exist and should be made explicit. *Box 9.7* provides a summary of the key points about the use of criteria to assess qualitative research raised in this chapter.

Box 9.7: Key points on 'criteria to assess qualitative research'

⌘ There is debate over whether it is feasible or appropriate to identify criteria to judge the quality of qualitative research. Perceptions of quality criteria are influenced by differing assumptions about the philosophical basis of qualitative research.

⌘ Perspectives range from complete rejection of the notion of criteria, to the application of alternative criteria specific to the qualitative paradigm, to those who advocate the use of quality criteria common to both quantitative and qualitative paradigms.

⌘ Many checklists, guidelines and criteria for assessing the quality of qualitative research exist, with a high proportion of them developed in medical or health services research. Most criteria attribute importance to validity, reliability and generalisability. However, the terminology used varies according to philosophical and methodological perspectives.

⌘ Consensus among qualitative researchers on language, terminology and notions of quality is important if the credibility of qualitative research is to be upheld. It is possible to identify pragmatic guidelines for 'good practice' in qualitative research in applied health research.

Acknowledgments

I would like to thank members of the Qualitative Research in Health Working Group at Liverpool School of Tropical Medicine (Helen Bromley, Grindl Dockery, Bertha Nhlema, Lois Orton, Sally Theobald and Rachel Tolhurst) for the many exhausting but enjoyable discussions about the nature of qualitative enquiry, and for their hard work in compiling our criteria for evaluating qualitative research.

References

Barbour RS (2001) Checklists for improving rigour in qualitative research: a case of the tail wagging the dog? *BMJ* **322**: 1115-7

Beck CT (1993) Qualitative research: the evaluation of its credibility, fittingness and auditability. *West J Nurs Res* **15**(2): 263-6

Blaxter M (1996) Criteria for qualitative research. *Med Sociol News* **22**: 68-71

Bryman A (1988) *Quantity and Quality in Social Research.* Unwin Hyman, London

Bryman A, Burgess RG, eds (1994) *Analysing Qualitative Data.* Routledge, London

Bush J, White M, Kai J, Rankin J, Bhopal R (2003) Understanding influences on smoking in Bangladeshi and Pakistani adults: community based, qualitative study. *BMJ* **326**: 962

Campbell R, Pound P, Pope C, Britten N, Pill R, Morgan M, Donovan J (2003) Evaluating meta-ethnography: a synthesis of qualitative research on lay experiences of diabetes and diabetes care. *Soc Sci Med* **56**(4): 671-84

Chapple A, Rogers A (1998) Explicit guidelines for qualitative research: a step in the right direction, a defence of the 'soft' option, or a form of sociological imperialism? *Fam Pract* **15**: 556-61

Cobb AJ, Hagemaster JN (1987) Ten criteria for evaluating qualitative research proposals. *J Nurs Educ* **26**(4): 138-43

Cook TD, Campbell, DT (1979) *Quasi-experimentation: Design Issues for Field Settings.* Rand MacNally, Chicago

Critical Appraisal Skills Programme (CASP) (2002)*10 Questions to Help You Make Sense of Qualitative Research.* CASP, Oxford

Department of Health (2003) Research Governance Framework [Online]. Available at: http://www.doh.gov.uk/research/rd3/nhsrandd/researchgovernance/govhome.htm [accessed 11 November, 2003]

Dixon-Woods M, Fitzpatrick R (2001) Qualitative research in systematic reviews. *Br Med J* **323**: 765-6

Elliot R, Fischer C, Rennie DL (1999) Evolving guidelines for publication of qualitative research studies in psychology and related fields. *Br J Clin Psychol* **38**(3): 215-29

Gahan C, Hannibal M (1999) *Doing Qualitative Research Using QSR NUD*IST.* Sage, London

Glaser BG, Strauss AL (1967) *The Discovery of Grounded Theory.* Aldine, Chicago

Greenhalgh T, Taylor R (1997) How to read a paper: papers that go beyond numbers (qualitative research). *Br Med J* **315**: 740–43

Hammersely D (1990) *Reading Ethnographic Research.* Longman, New York

Hammersley M (1992) *What's Wrong with Ethnography?* Routledge, London

Kirk J, Miller M (1986) *Reliability and Validity in Qualitative Research.* Sage, Newbury Park, CA

Kuckartz U (2002) WinMAX software. Germany: VERBI Software-Consult-Research GmbH Berlin

Le Compte, M Goetz J (1982) Problems of reliability and validity in ethnographic research. *Rev Educational Res* **52**(1): 31–60

Leininger M (1994) Evaluation criteria and critique of qualitative research studies. In: Morse JM, ed. *Critical Issues in Qualitative Research Methods.* Sage, Thousand Oaks, CA

Lincoln Y, Guba E (1985) *Naturalisitc Inquiry.* Sage, Beverly Hills

Malterud K (2001) Qualitative research: standards, challenges and guidelines. *The Lancet* **358**: 483–88

Mays N, Pope C (1995) Qualitative research: rigour and qualitative research. *Br Med J* **311**: 109–12

Mays N, Pope C (2000) Quality in qualitative health research. In Pope C, Mays N, eds. *Qualitative Research in Healthcare.* BMJ Books, London

Miles MB, Huberman AM (1994) *Qualitative Data Analysis: An expanded source book.* Sage, London

Murphy E, Dingwall R, Greatbatch D, Parker S, Watson P (1998) Qualitative research methods in health technology assessment. *Health Technol Assess* **2**(16)

Murphy D, Pope L, Frost J (2003) Women's views on the impact of operative delivery in the second stage of labour: qualitative study interview. *Br Med J* **327**: 1132–35

Murray S (2000) Relation between private sector health insurance and high rates of Caesarean section in Chile: qualitative and quantitative study. *Br Med J* **321**: 1501–5

Nhlema B, Kemp J, Steenbergen S, Theobald S, Tang S, Squire SB (2003) *A Systematic Analysis of TB and Poverty, Technical Paper, Stop TB partnership*. World Health Organization, Geneva

Popay J, Rogers A, Williams G (1998) Qualitative research and evidence-based healthcare. *J Roy Soc Med* **191**(35): 32–7

Qualitative Research in Health Working Group (QRHWG) (2002) Criteria for evaluating qualitative research. [Online]. Available online: http://www.liv.ac.uk/lstm/QRMweb/QRHWG.htm [9 September 2003]

Ritchie J, Spencer L (1994) Qualitative data analysis for applied policy research. In: Bryman A, Burgess RB, eds. *Analysing Qualitative Data*. Routledge, London

Sandelowski M (1986) The problem of rigour in qualitative research. *Adv Nursing Sci* **8**: 27–37

Silverman D (1989) Telling convincing stories: a plea for cautious positivism in case studies. In: Glasner B, Moreno JD, eds. *The Qualitative-quantitative Distinction in the Social Sciences*. Kluwer Academic Publishers, Dordrecht

Smith J (1984) The problem of criteria for judging interpretive enquiry. *Educational Evaluation and Policy Analysis* **6**: 379–91

Spencer L, Ritchie J, Lewis J, Dillon L (2003) Quality in qualitative evaluation: a framework for assessing research evidence. Government Chief Social Researcher's Office, Occasional Papers Series No.2. Cabinet Office, London

Stapleton H, Kirkham M, Thomas G (2002) Qualitative study of evidence-based leaflets in maternity care. *Br Med J* **324**: 639

Treloar C, Champness S, Simpson P, Higginbotham N (2000) Critical appraisal checklist for qualitative research studies. *Indian J Pediatr* **67**(5): 347–51

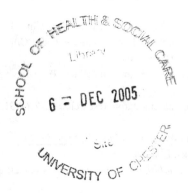

Index